THE CRUNCH FITNESS GUIDES

BEGINNER'S LUCK

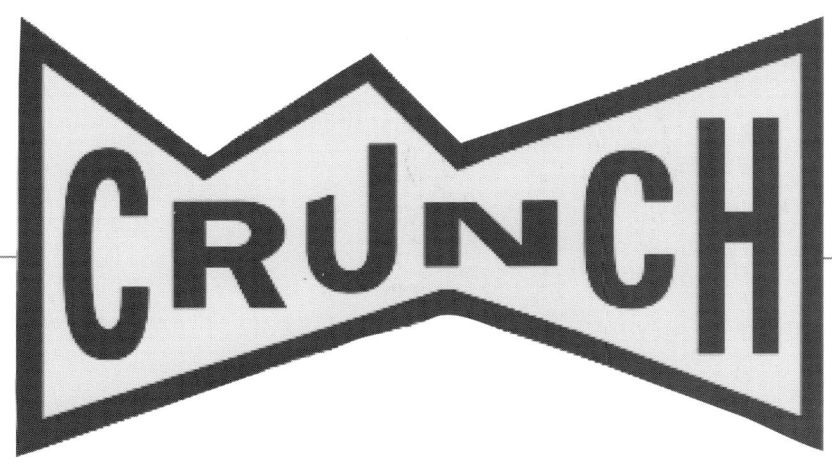

HATHERLEIGH
NEW YORK

GetFitNow.com Books
An Independent Imprint of Hatherleigh Press

Copyright © 1999 by Crunch Fitness

All rights reserved. No part of this book may be reproduced in any form or by any means, electronic or mechanical, including photocopying, recording, or by any information storage or retrieval system, without permission in writing from the publisher.

GetFitNow.com Books
An Independent Imprint of Hatherleigh Press
an affiliate of W.W. Norton & Company
500 Fifth Avenue
New York, NY 10110
1-800-367-2550
www.getfitnow.com

Before beginning any strenuous exercise program consult your physician. The author and publisher of this book and workout disclaim any liability, personal or professional, resulting from the misapplication of any of the training procedures described in this publication.

All GetFitNow.com books are available for bulk purchase, special promotions, and premiums. For more information, please contact the manager of our Special Sales department at 1-800-367-2550.

Library of Congress Cataloging in-Publication Data

Crunch Fitness,
    Beginner's luck / Crunch.
      p.   cm. — (The Crunch Fitness Series)
    ISBN 1-57826-027-2 (alk. paper)
    1. Exercise. 2. Physical fitness. 3. Weight training equipment and supplies.
  I. Crunch. II. Series.
  RA781.B3936 1999
  613.7—cc21   99-34884
                                                                                                                        CIP

Series Editor: Heather Ogilvie
Cover design: Lisa Fyfe
Text design and composition: John Reinhardt Book Design
Photographs: Peter Field Peck with Canon® cameras and lenses on Fuji® print and slide film

Printed in Canada on acid-free paper

10 9 8 7 6 5 4 3 2 1

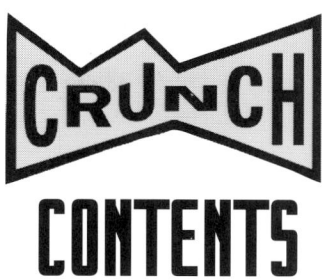

CONTENTS

Introduction to Crunch Fitness Guides v

Acknowledgments vii

PART 1
Fitness in the Misinformation Age   1

PART 2
What's Your Motivation?   11

PART 3
The Workout   17

PART 4
Your Fitness Log   77

Crunch Locations 135

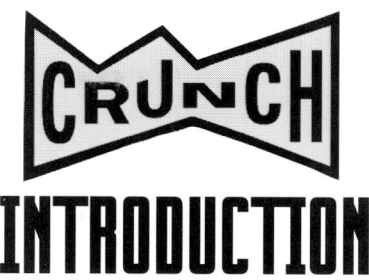

INTRODUCTION

Welcome to CRUNCH! For over a decade, we've been welcoming people of all shapes, sizes, ages, and fitness levels to our gyms. As we've expanded from a tiny, one-room aerobics studio in New York's East Village to cities across the country (and even to Tokyo), we've offered group fitness classes, personal training, and equipment to appeal to everyone from stressed-out workaholics and jet setters to senior citizens and expectant moms. We're living up to our motto, "No Judgements!"

We're aware that some people shy away from joining a gym or from starting a fitness program because they think it demands too great a change in their lifestyle. But at CRUNCH, we believe you shouldn't have to change your lifestyle in order to be fit. In fact, we believe your workout should change to fit your lifestyle. It is our firm belief that the success of a fitness program has nothing to do with how many hours you spend in the gym, but how good you feel when you're outside the gym, living your life.

That's why we've created these fitness guides—to show you that no matter what your lifestyle, there's a workout you can do that will complement it and get you fit. For example, we designed the *Road Warrior Workout* for people who spend a lot of time traveling on business. These folks don't have to give up their fitness programs—in fact, by doing a workout specially adapted to life on the road, they can maintain their fitness level and become less susceptible to all the common aches and discomforts of travel.

Get Fit in a CRUNCH is for those people who are trying to shape up in time for a big event—a wedding, a reunion, a trip to the beach. Based on CRUNCH's popular class, Emergency Beach Training, *Get Fit in a CRUNCH* lays out a safe, effective four-week workout, 12-week workout, and six-month workout.

Since the hardest part of any fitness program is starting it, we've

INTRODUCTION

written *Beginner's Luck* to help people stay motivated and become more familiar with—and less intimidated by—basic cardiovascular and strength training exercises. It's a workout you can take at your own pace, according to your own goals.

Look for additions to the CRUNCH Fitness Guides targeting time-pressed workaholics, first-time marathon runners, and people who want to eliminate or avoid common back pain and improve posture.

At CRUNCH, we don't want you to conform to some workout fad or a lifestyle of spending more time at the gym than at play. We want to give you workout options that will conform to your lifestyle—without judgement.

Doug Levine
Founder and CEO
Crunch Fitness International, Inc.
www.crunch.com

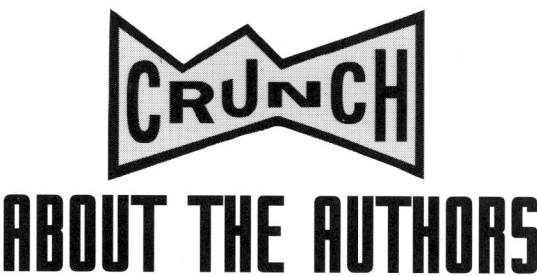

ABOUT THE AUTHORS

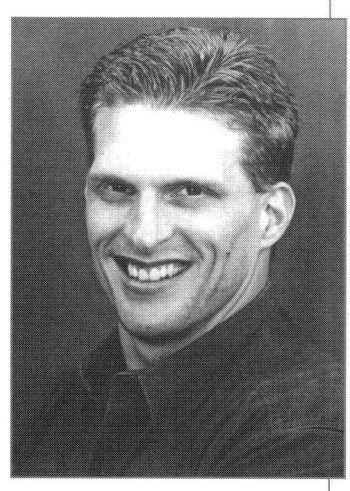

Brad Hamler, a fitness professional in new York City who has worked at several CRUNCH gyms, designed the Beginner's Luck workout.

Brad is originally from Ohio, where he began his career in fitness. He was a nationally ranked Natural Competitive Bodybuilder, and he has appeared in various fitness and bodybuilding publications. In addition to a B.A. in Business Administration from Findlay University, Brad has earned the following professional credentials: Master Trainer from the National Academy of Sports Medicine (NASM), Certified Personal Trainer (ACE), and Post-Rehab Conditioning Specialist (AAHFP).

In 1994, Brad started his own company, Hamler Fitness Team, an in-house personal training business. Today, Brad teaches classes such as Ultimate Conditioning, Abdominals Core Training, and Cardio-Conditioning. He lectures and regularly holds seminars on golf and fitness as well as other fitness topics.

Brad's other passions include his four-year-old daughter, Katja, and golf.

ABOUT THE AUTHORS

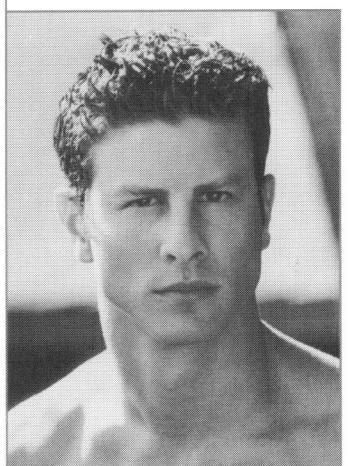

Brian Delmonico designed the stretching routine for *Beginner's Luck*. A trainer in CRUNCH's 13th Street gym in New York City, Brian began his career as a gymnast at age 6. In his teens, he was on the National Gymnastics Team for three years, and he's a three-time All-American and two-time Big Ten Champion. He graduated from Ohio State University with a Bachelor's Degree in Education and Nutrition. Brian is certified by the USGF in Safety and Stretching—and he has a black belt in Tae Kwon Do.

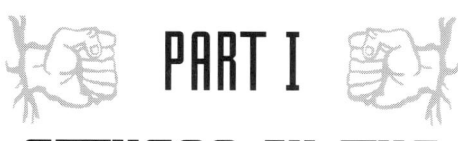

PART I
FITNESS IN THE MISINFORMATION AGE

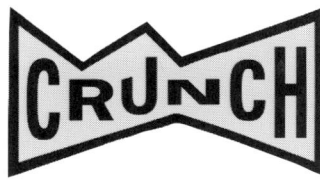

When it comes to sticking with a fitness program, beginners need all the luck they can get. Statistics suggest that 50% of all people who begin an exercise program drop out within the first six months. If lifetime fitness is your goal (and it should be), the odds are stacked against you.

Consider this: Today, 20 years since the fitness revolution in this country began, Americans are fatter and have more fitness-related injuries than ever before. Some revolution! Shouldn't we be leaner, healthier, and more energetic? What went wrong?

Too little good information has been lost in a pool of misinformation—misinformation we're all too willing to embrace as truth. We've got a leap-before-you-look culture. If the media says, "Everyone's aerobicizing," we run out and join an aerobics class. If marketers say, "Everyone's got a Soloflex machine at home," we run out and buy one. If ads tell us to "just do it," well, we're likely to just overdo it.

That's because we Americans like quick fixes. In the age of microwaves and Pay-Per-View, we embrace anything that promises results quickly with a minimum of effort. Then, when those results don't come as quickly as we expected, we drop that program and get with the next one that comes along. It may be a Jane Fonda video one week, yoga the next, kickboxing the next, until we're exhausted, frustrated, injured, and less likely than ever to stick with a fitness program.

The truth is, a person could have tried all these exercise programs and still essentially be a beginner when it comes to fitness. Why? Because despite all the exercising, that person never really understood what the particular fitness program could and could not do. And just as important, she didn't understand what her own fitness goals were and whether that particular exercise program was the best way to accomplish them.

There may be nothing wrong with a lot of the exercise fads that are out there. What's wrong is a typical beginner's approach to them as well as his or her expectations. So how do you avoid such frustration and begin a life-long fitness program you can really stick with?

First, you have to clear your head of all the unrealistic promises marketers have pitched to you over the years. You must be willing to spend a little time learning the basic facts about your body and what exercise can and can't do. And finally, you have write down some realistic goals and a plan for achieving them. In this book, we're going to help you do all those things. Your beginner's odds just got a whole lot better.

TRUTH OR CONSEQUENCES

Bombarded with so many ads for home exercise equipment as well as images of impossibly buff celebrities and athletes, it's no wonder most Americans harbor many myths and misconceptions about what constitutes exercise. Let's look at 12 of the biggest misconceptions that sabotage most people's fitness routines.

Misconception #1:
You have to live at the gym to be successful.

Truth: Yes, if you want to look the way Linda Hamilton did in *Terminator 2*, then you have to spend about six hours a day at the gym. But can you afford to? Are you really that motivated? After all, she was paid handsomely to spend all that time working out, which was probably a big part of her motivation.

But do *you* have to spend that much time at the gym to be successful? Not if your definition of success is to maintain good physical fitness. You need only about one hour, a few days a week. But you do need to make that commitment.

Misconception #2:
The more you work out, the more fit you'll be.

Truth: If you saw the same people at the gym seven days a week, for two or three hours a day, you know what you'd think? That these people are *not* healthy! And you'd be right.

That's because your body needs rest. You should *always* set one day a week aside and rest. In other words, do not exercise on that day! Furthermore, and equally important, *never* work out the same muscle group two days in a row. If you're doing ab crunches every single day—stop! Doing so defeats the purpose of strength training—you won't tone your muscles, you'll injure them.

Misconception #3:
You can turn fat into muscle.

Truth: Just as medieval alchemists could not turn iron into gold, you cannot turn fat into muscle. They are two completely different substances. However, you can burn fat and get rid of it by exercising. As you shed the fat that's been obscuring your muscles, you then start to see your muscles. You don't really gain muscle just by strength training. You improve your muscles' "tone," or appearance, because all that fat's no longer in the way!

It sounds brutal, but each time you work out with weights, you cause little "traumas" or tears in your muscles as they are forced to work more than usual. But these little traumas are easily repaired when you sleep. And where your muscle has rebuilt itself, it actually becomes stronger.

Of course, the trick is to work out so that you create these little traumas, but not major traumas. Remember, the most effective workout is a safe one. If you really injure yourself, you can't exercise at all, which obviously isn't very effective.

Misconception #4:
Your body changes its physical appearance at the gym.

Truth: Your body changes when it repairs itself—at night, when you're asleep. You may notice some increase in muscle size right after a workout, but that will disappear—fortunately or unfortunately, depending on whether you want to "bulk up"—within a couple of hours.

Again, this highlights the importance of rest. If you don't give your body a chance to recuperate, you'll never see any beneficial results of your workout.

Misconception #5:
Working out with weights will make you "big."

Truth: Women often avoid weight training because they don't want to develop large muscles. As a result, their fitness program is unbalanced, they don't reach their fitness goals, they are more prone to injury, and they waste a lot of energy on ineffective and inefficient workouts.

The truth is, unless a woman takes steroids or works out more than six hours a day, she is *not* going to develop the musculature that a man would, given the same amount of weight training. Women's hormones—or lack of certain hormones—prevents women from developing large muscles.

WHEN IS THE BEST TIME TO WORK OUT?

The best time is the most convenient time—in other words, the time you will actually do it. Statistics suggest, however, that beginners who work out first thing in the morning stick with their fitness programs longer than beginners who schedule their workouts at other times.

However, by avoiding weight training entirely, women are missing out on its many benefits. These include increased strength, stronger bones (and less risk of developing osteoporosis), reduced risk of injury to joints and muscles during any activity, improved cardiovascular fitness, and more efficient (i.e., less time-consuming) overall training.

Misconception #6:
The best way to test your fitness level is to get on the scale.

Truth: Weight is not the best indicator of overall health. You can be the same height and age as the next person, but weigh more—yet be perfectly healthy. That's because you could have larger, denser bones—which you do not want to lose! Losing weight may not be in your best interest. Maybe you can't be too rich, but you definitely can be too thin.

Some experts will tell you the best fitness test is a body fat test, which precisely measures the percentage of fat on your body. This test can be done only at certain gyms, clinics, and universities.

But that's not necessarily the best test of fitness. The best fitness test is how you feel and how you look. The best equipment: a full-length mirror. It will tell you everything you need to know. The key is to try to look at your body as objectively as possible. (Just look from the neck down.) As you progress on your fitness program, notice how your body starts to change. Record what you notice in a training log.

The second best test is the "peer" test. You have passed this test when one of your friends says, "Did you lose weight?" or "Did you cut your hair?"

Misconception #7:
Spot reduction exercises work.

Truth: There is only one spot reduction technique that works, and it's called *liposuction*.

Spot reduction exercises waste time and energy. But they sure are tempting! Who wants to work out all their muscles if they want to lose weight only on their thighs or stomach? Why not just do crunches for half an hour? Or work out on the Stairmaster for 40 minutes?

There's a very good reason: Your body is smarter than that. Your body sees that same, dull workout coming every time. So instead of working out those poor thigh muscles for 30 minutes, your body is going to recruit energy from all the underused muscle groups that could possibly pitch in to help. (Bear in mind, your body always chooses the path of least resistance.)

But if you were working out all the different muscle groups, it would not be so easy for your body to enlist the help of other peripheral muscles, now fatigued, when an exercise really focuses on one group. Thus, thorough weight training actually helps you isolate the function of each muscle, including the one you most want to tone. A thorough body workout makes the time you spend on each muscle group more effective than a "spot-reduction" workout. That means you can actually spend less time working out to get the results you want.

Another thing to consider is that the body burns fat as fuel from wherever it is most convenient for the body to do so—not necessarily from where you want it to. That means that if you work out on the Stairmaster in hopes of losing fat from your thighs, your body may actually decide it's easier to burn the fat around your stomach first. In other words, targeting one area is no guarantee that that's where you will lose the fat first.

Furthermore, by focusing on one muscle group to the exclusion of all others, you will end up with muscle imbalances, leaving the weaker muscles and joints more susceptible to injury.

A good fitness program works out all the major muscle groups—be wary of any program or equipment that touts limited workouts or spot reduction.

Misconception #8:
For an exercise to be effective, you have to "feel it."

Truth: So many people push themselves too far, believing in the adage, "No pain, no gain." This misguided belief has led to countless injuries. The truth is, feelings can be deceptive. Feeling one muscle really work may not be an indication of the *quality* of the exercise, especially if you've worked that muscle too hard or incorrectly.

Misconception #9:
If you're not losing weight—or if you're actually gaining weight—you're not making progress.

Truth: Let's say you're 130 pounds and you want to weigh 120. You start working out, and after a couple of weeks you notice your weight has actually gone up to 132! What gives?

Well, this happens quite often, and unfortunately, most beginners in this situation throw in the towel and quit their exercise program.

What a waste! The truth is, muscle tissue, which increases its density slightly as it repairs itself after a workout, weighs more than fat tissue. In other words, muscles are more dense than fat. So for a brief time, you could be losing fat, but gaining weight—in the form of more toned muscles. This is *not* the time to quit. Eventually, if you have fat to lose, you will lose weight!

The trick is not to be scale conscious. Unfortunately, telling an American not to be scale conscious is like telling a dog to give up a bone. Instead of jumping on the scale twice a day, ask yourself: How do I *feel*? Do I feel better? If you feel better, your fitness program is working, and you will eventually *see* the results as well as feel them.

Misconception #10:
Through proper diet and exercise, you can lose 10 pounds or more a week.

Truth: No doubt about it, you can lose ten pounds in one week. But if you do, it won't be through proper (meaning healthy) diet and exercise. In fact, to be healthy, you should *never lose more than two pounds a week*, no matter how overweight you are. Yes, that sounds like slow going. But you should make a commitment to fitness for life, not just until your wedding, or until the summer, or until your high school reunion.

Don't hurt your body—make it the best it can be. If you lose more than two pounds a week, you're setting yourself up for rebounding, which is very traumatic for your body. Remember, your goal is to achieve a consistent level of health and fitness. Yo-yo dieting and exercising is *not* healthy.

Misconception #11:
Most gym members work out at least once a week.

Truth: Out of 365 opportunities—opportunities a member pays for, mind you—the typical gym member shows up only *four times a year*. Not even once a month! Considering the cost of membership, those are four pretty expensive visits!

Some people join gyms because they figure the cost will give them an extra incentive to work out. But this rationale rarely works. Just think how many people buy expensive clothes or nifty kitchen appliances that just sit in the closet unworn or unused.

Face it, lots of people—usually right after New Year's or right before summer—sign up at the gym, go once or twice, then drop out. Why? Because they haven't really made a firm commitment to staying fit. They haven't defined their goals. They did it just because it seemed like the thing to do.

But if you don't have a reason, realistic goals, and commitment, you will fail. For instance, would you sign up to take a course in Russian if you didn't plan to go to Russia, read books in Russian, or communicate with Russian friends or relatives?

The first step in any fitness program is setting a goal and making a commitment to it. Put it in writing. And come to terms with obstacles that may prevent you from achieving your goals. For instance:

Lifetime Goal: To achieve consistent physical fitness over the course of my life and improve the quality of my life.
Long-Term Goal: To spend one hour a day, six days a week on a workout that combines flexibility, strength, and cardiovascular training.
Short-Term Goals: On three non-consecutive days, jog for 20 minutes at my target heart rate. On two non-consecutive days, do one set of weight training exercises. Hold all stretches for at least 10 seconds.
Obstacles to overcome: Wake up one hour earlier. Buy new running shoes. Buy a set of dumbbells (or join local gym).

Keeping a fitness log of your goals and obstacles—and checking off whether you've met them each week—will help motivate you. You'll be able to chart your progress and see how working out is improving your life.

BEGINNER'S LUCK

Misconception #12:
Fitness professionals and personal trainers are only for celebrities and athletes.

Truth: Let's say you want to play golf or tennis. Maybe you've played a few times with a friend. But you know that if you really want to learn to play, you need to take lessons from a golf or tennis pro.

Well, lots of people decide to work out, but rarely do they think they need a fitness professional to show them how to do it. Surrounded by more equipment than you can shake a nine iron at, people still assume they can figure out how to use it all properly. Just watch the person on the machine before you, right?

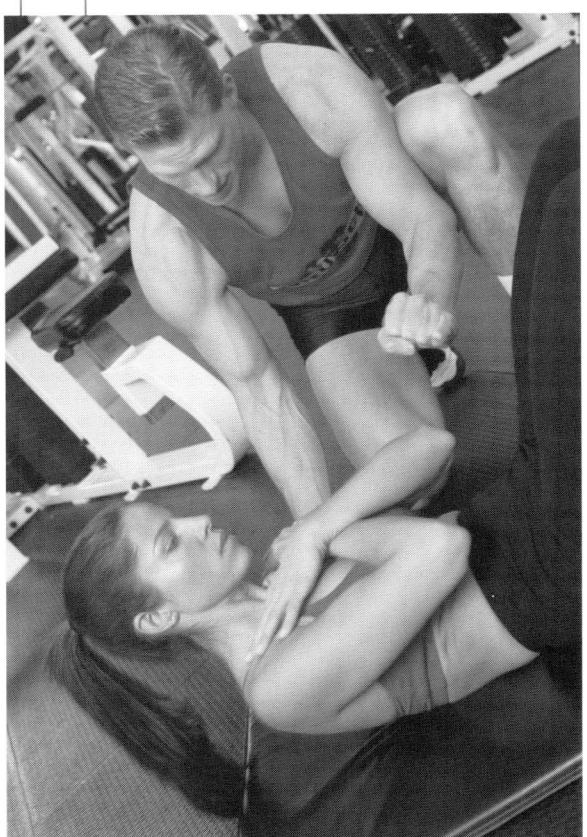

Well, it's not so simple. Without any training, some folks are liable to get on a machine and hurt themselves and then BAM!—that ends their expensive gym membership. Or they use the machines incorrectly and don't get as effective a workout as they could.

The fact is, if you can afford a gym membership, hiring a fitness professional is often a good investment—a pro will help make sure you're going to get the most out of your membership. That's not to say that you always need a fitness professional every time you work out, or that you will always need a fitness professional for the rest of your days. But they can be especially helpful to beginners, and they are definitely not just for celebrities and athletes.

Of course, not all fitness professionals are good ones. By reading the fitness facts in this book, you'll know to be suspicious if a pro makes outrageous promises ("You will lose 10 pounds in one week!")

FITNESS IN THE MISINFORMATION AGE

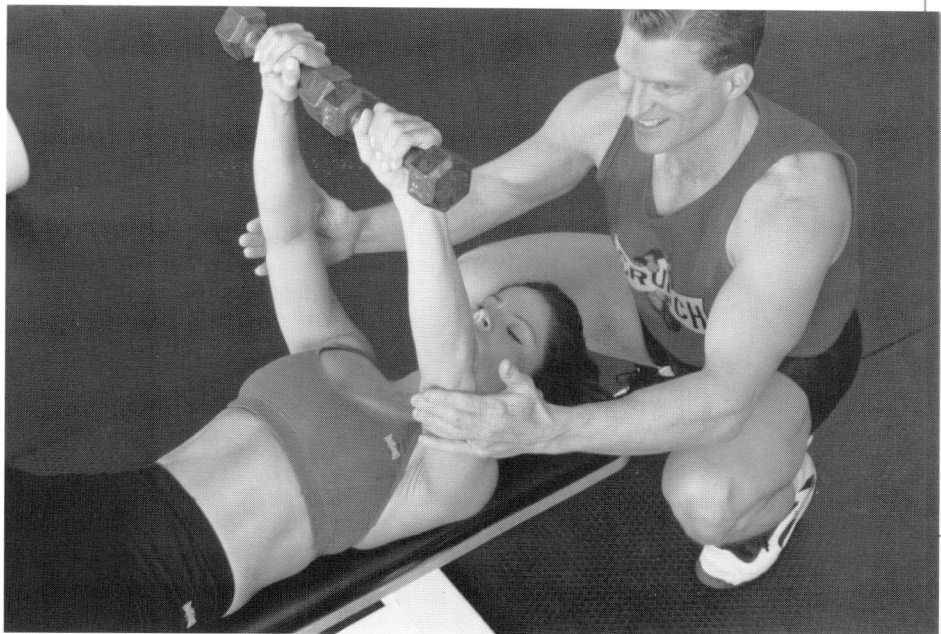

or gives you false information ("You should just work out your abs because that's where you want to lose weight").

It's important to choose a fitness professional who really listens to you and understands your goals. Some fitness professionals think all their clients' goals are the same: peak (read "Olympic") physical condition. But not every client wants to compete in a triathalon. Not every client has more than an hour a day to devote to training. Most people just want to feel and look good. They want good physical fitness.

Consider this: What's the first thing you think about when you get up in the morning? Maybe you think, "What do I have to do today at work?" "What chores do I have to do?" "When am I going to spend time with my spouse or kids?"

Well, the first thing a fitness professional usually asks when he or she wakes up is, "When am I going to work out today?" Because a pro may have different personal fitness goals than most of his or her clients, sometimes even great pros can lose sight of their clients' goals. So don't be afraid to remind your fitness professional about your own personal fitness goals.

Finally, bear in mind that you don't have to hire a personal trainer or even join a gym to achieve consistent physical fitness. After all, the best fitness program of all is the one you will do—and if getting to or affording a gym isn't convenient for you, a membership alone will not make you fit.

BEGINNER'S LUCK

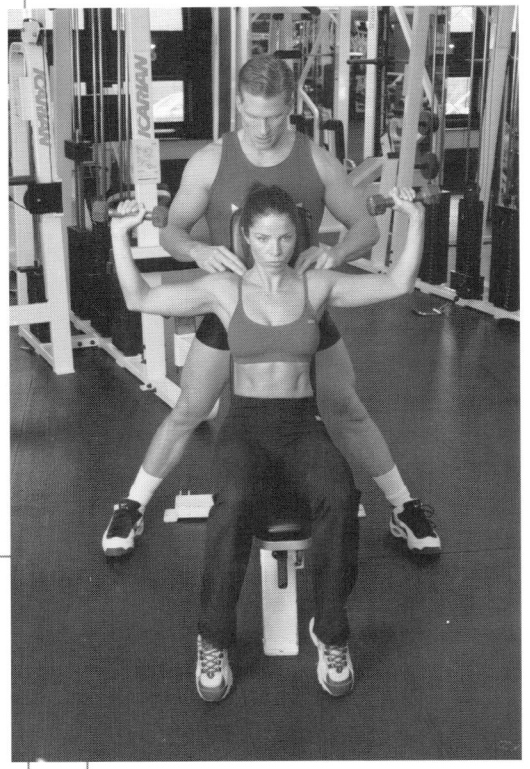

Some of the exercises in this book's workout use gym equipment and describe how to use the equipment properly. That's because those beginners who choose to work out at a gym should know how to take advantage of the equipment that's there. Equipment can be intimidating, so our workout describes the proper use of common gym machines and equipment. But for every equipment exercise, there is also a similar exercise you can do without equipment. For example, when working your leg muscles, doing squats can be just as effective as using the leg press equipment.

While gym equipment can be intimidating to beginners, beginners actually benefit most from using it. That's because the equipment helps "program" your muscles to do the exercises correctly, within a limited range of motion. When you do a free-standing exercise, your body has a greater chance of going outside the most effective range of motion as it tries to maintain its balance. In that respect, gym equipment offers an easier and safer way to work specific muscles.

That is not to say, however, that you can't hurt yourself on a piece of equipment, so read our exercise descriptions carefully! And choose a place to work out based on your lifestyle and what is most convenient for you.

PART II
WHAT'S YOUR MOTIVATION?

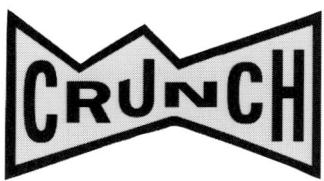

Many beginners fail to stick to their workout program for four simple reasons:

1. They haven't made a firm commitment to working out because they don't know why they're doing it ("everyone else is doing it" isn't a reason).
2. They haven't written down what their workout is going to be.
3. They overdo their workout in the first week, injure themselves, and hang up their gym shorts for good.
4. They underdo their workout, and when they fail to see results, they quit.

Regarding the first reason for failure, answer this multiple choice question: "Why do I want to start a fitness program?"

(a) Because I want to look like Arnold (or Madonna).
(b) Because I want to lose weight and look better.
(c) Because I want to feel better, improve the quality of my life, and maintain a consistent level of physical condition over the course of my lifetime.
(d) Because I want to meet people at the gym and be seen in my designer sweats.

If you answered (a), get a grip. If you start a fitness program with that goal, you are most likely going to fail. Unless, of course, you are willing to devote six hours a day to the gym and do so for as long as you want to look so buff. Unless you are an elite athlete or in the entertainment industry, such a goal is probably not realistic for you. And in trying too hard to achieve it, you may end up hurting yourself more than helping yourself. Consider the nutritionists, sports doctors, trainers, masseuses, plastic surgeons, make-up artists, etc. that celebrities hire to help them avoid and treat injuries ... Can you really afford all that?

TIPS FOR STAYING MOTIVATED

1. **Start with small goals that lead to larger goals.** For example, a small goal may be to jog continuously for 20 minutes two days this week. A larger goal is to be able to jog for 35 minutes three days a week by the end of six weeks. As you accomplish easier goals, you'll be encouraged to keep working toward larger ones.
2. **Set attainable goals.** "Losing 50 pounds in one month" is not a realistic goal. Again, start small.
3. **Reward yourself when you attain your goals.** For instance, go to the movies or out to dinner or buy yourself a new dress.
4. **Keep a training log.** A log will chart your progress and highlight problems you may need to address.
5. **Take periodic photos.** The camera doesn't lie. Once a month, paste a photo of yourself in your training log. While you may notice small changes every week, a monthly photo will show just how far you've come. And remember to look—really *look*—at your body in a full-length mirror periodically. You'll see the changes.
6. **Think positively.** Think of yourself as healthy and fit. Your attitude can go a long way toward achieving your goals. Visualize yourself as an athlete, as strong and energetic.
7. **Listen to your body.** The better you feel and look, the more tempted you may be to overdo it. When your muscles start to ache more than usual, if you suffer from insomnia or unusual fatigue, you could be overdoing it. Lower the intensity of your workout for a while.

If you answered (b), you're like most people. The trouble is, these folks become overly *scale conscious*. That means that the only way they measure their progress is in pounds. They don't pay attention to other benefits of a fitness program, and when they reach their weight goal, they quit exercising—and then the pounds return. This scale-conscious approach to fitness leads to "yo-yo" training and dieting that is definitely not in your body's best interest.

If you answered (c), congratulations! You are ready to start—and stick to—an exercise program. Repeat your goals like a mantra: "I want to feel better, improve the quality of my life, and maintain my peak physical condition. I want to feel better, improve the quality...." At the end of every week, ask yourself just that: How do I feel? How has the quality of my life improved? By tracking your responses, you'll be surprised how much progress you've made toward achieving true fitness. And, you'll have a continuous source of motivation.

If you answered (d), you do not have the commitment to really benefit from a workout program. You may achieve your goals of attracting attention, but it may not be the kind of attention you really want. After all, most of the people who are seriously committed to working out at the gym aren't there for your reasons.

Remember this: **Being committed to a fitness program is not about what you do in the gym (or what you wear at the gym), but how you feel outside the gym.**

WHAT IS PROGRESS?

Beginners who get through the first two months of a fitness program are likely to stick with that program. Why? Because at no other point during training is a person likely to experience as much progress. What kind of progress? You will notice your body getting leaner, you will fit better in your clothes, you will sleep better at night, you will have more energy during the day, you will, overall, *feel* better.

Reality check: That doesn't necessarily mean you will lose 20 pounds in two weeks—get that idea right out of your head! For one thing, every person's body is a little different and will lose weight at its own rate. Second, losing more than two pounds a week is *never* healthy—and achieving and maintaining good health is your goal. Repeat after me: *Achieving and maintaining good health is my goal.*

What about tracking your progress after those first few months of working out? What exactly is progress? What should you look for? When you feel great, what's the next step?

Maintaining a consistent level of physical fitness is that next "step." That's right, maintaining fitness is actually progress. Why is that? As we age, our metabolism (the rate at which our cells grow and our tissues heal) naturally slows down—to compensate for that natural decline, we have to work harder to maintain a consistent level of fitness.

BEGINNER'S LUCK

If you reach a fitness level where you are happy with how you feel, and then you stop exercising, you'll be surprised how quickly your body reverts back to a sluggish, unfit condition. So not seeing signs of progress doesn't mean that you're not making any! Maintaining a consistent level of fitness *is* progress—and an achievement to be proud of.

After your beginning phase during which you see and feel the most dramatic changes, you will enter the maintenance phase, or, as some fitness professionals like to call it, the "keep-on-keeping-on" phase. At this phase, you won't experience dramatic changes. But to keep your body from hitting a "training plateau," you may need to juggle your workout a little and give your body some new exercises to adapt to. Again, the signs of progress will be how consistently good you feel, rather than any dramatic changes in your size or shape.

After the keep-on-keeping-on phase comes the dedicated athlete phase. This phase involves making the journey—that last 5 to 10% of the way—to your maximum physical potential. This is the point where you must have inspiration by the boatload and the time and dedication to make every minute you spend in the gym a challenge. If you fit this profile, you probably were offered several million dollars to star opposite Bruce Willis in an action film. Or to play for the Houston Rockets. Or maybe you have an addiction to extreme sports. In any case, if you make it to the place where you want to travel that last 5% of the way, then this is the point where you need to buy a different fitness book . . .

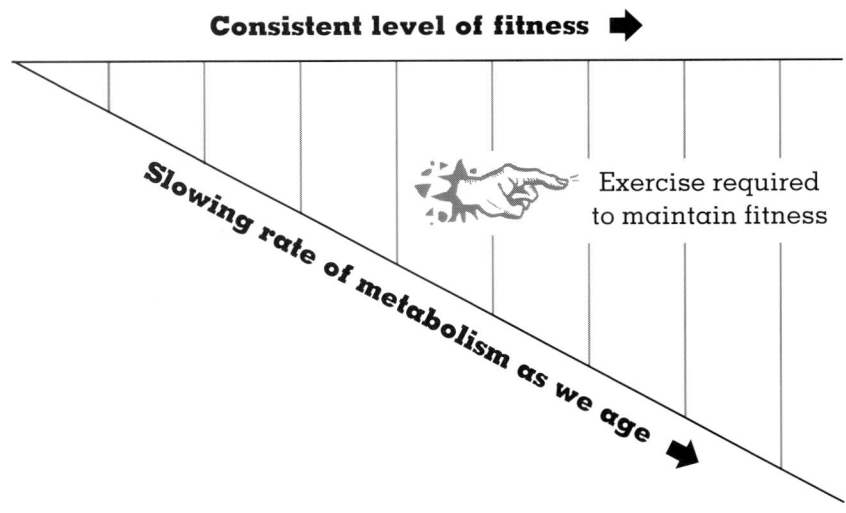

WHAT'S YOUR MOTIVATION?

EXCUSES, EXCUSES

Nothing sabotages your fitness program more than creating excuses not to exercise. You may think your excuses are perfectly valid. But considering what they're robbing you of—looking and feeling great, being healthier and more energetic, possibly living longer, and enjoying a better quality of life—maybe your excuses are not so acceptable.

MORE REASONS TO WORK OUT

Besides looking better and slimmer, working out can help you to:

1. Enhance quality of life
2. Reduce stress
3. Relieve depression
4. Become stronger
5. Increase endurance for sports, dancing, and other activities
6. Prevent heart disease and osteoporosis

Once you see what the workout entails, you'll say, "Heck, I can do that!" It's not that difficult. The trick is to motivate yourself to do it regularly and realize the folly of your excuses.

Let's take a good hard look at two of the most common excuses people make not to work out on any given day:

I don't have time. Of course you work hard and have to have some time left over for family and friends and sleep. But how often do you spend an hour at the mall or an hour watching sit-coms or an hour hitting the snooze button every ten minutes in the morning? Is that time really well spent?

If you want something badly enough, you always make time for it. The key to making time for working out is to *schedule your workouts*. Write them—in pen—in your date book. Another key is to schedule them *at the same time every day*. If you do this, there will come a time when you actually look forward to your daily workout.

Another key is not to think of your workout as a chore. Think of it as something you're doing for yourself. This is time you have to yourself, to clear your head, and to focus on just you.

I'm too tired. Energy begets energy. It's a paradox: Expending energy by exercising gives you more energy. That's one reason why it's better to work out early in the morning rather than late at night. After a workout, chances are you won't be exhausted, you'll actually be energized or "pumped."

Another benefit of working out is that when you do sleep, you will sleep better. Regular exercise promotes deep, restful sleep. If you're currently tired all the time, it's probably because the sleep you're getting isn't very deep or restful.

Finally, when you do skip a workout, don't berate yourself. Don't convince yourself that one missed workout is a sign of failure and that you should just quit for good. You will have setbacks. And you may not reach all of your goals in the time you give yourself. But if you get right back into your program as soon as you can, you'll find that your successes will add up more quickly than your setbacks.

While exercising can be fun and energizing and even addictive, working out is work. Some days you're just not going to be motivated. Pushing yourself through those times will be hard, but your sense of accomplishment afterwards will be enormous. Remind yourself why you're doing it. Focus on your achievements and plan to reward yourself for reaching periodic goals.

Just getting yourself to the gym, even when you so don't feel like working out, sends a positive message of consistency to yourself. The days you don't quite feel up to par, go for an easy workout rather than no workout at all. An easy workout is better than no workout. Blowing it off altogether on just one day can quickly lead to a downward spiral of missed workouts—and eventually no fitness program at all.

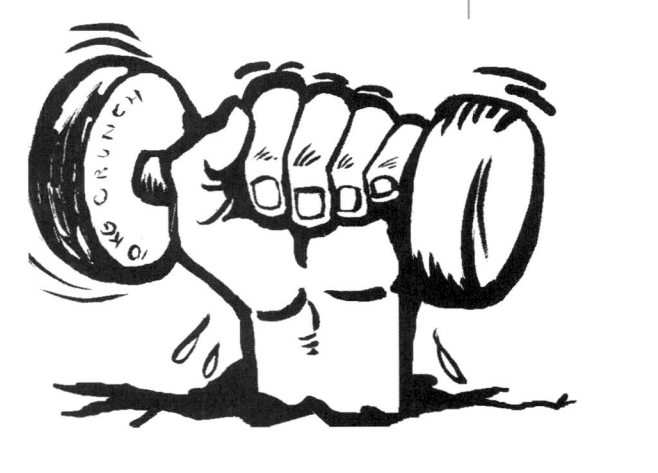

PART III
THE WORKOUT

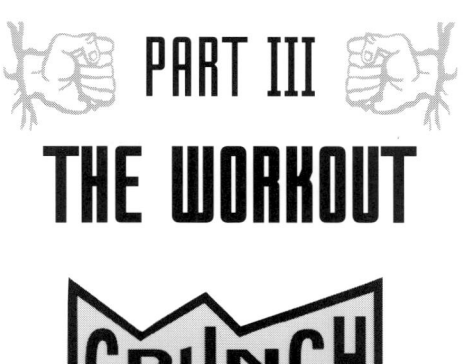

Beginners should set aside one hour a day, three days a week for their fitness program. There is no reason why you shouldn't be able to achieve your goal of consistent physical fitness by devoting this small amount of time to exercise. If you need more than an hour a day, six days a week, chances are you are not exercising as efficiently as you could. Unless you want to be a world-class athlete and supermodel like Gabrielle Reese, you do not need to spend hours every day in the gym. The workout we're going to describe is designed to be very efficient, so that you're done quickly yet get great results.

Always rest one day a week. That's the time your body repairs itself—and that's when all the improvements occur. If you don't give your body a day of rest, you won't be giving it a chance to improve!

All good workouts have three main components: cardiovascular training, strength training, and flexibility training. To ignore one component and focus on, say, just cardio training is not only inefficient (meaning you'll have to stay on that treadmill a whole lot longer to experience as much improvement), but it can also lead to fitness imbalances: If one part of your body (say, your leg muscles) are more toned than other muscles, you may actually be more prone to injuries in the long term.

Strength training. As we discussed in Chapter 1, many people, especially women, have gross misconceptions about strength (weight) training. Working out a few days a week with dumbbells or body bars is *not* going to give you bulging Olympic muscles! It will tone your muscles, make your muscles *and* your bones stronger, and reduce your risk of injury.

BEGINNER'S LUCK

Misconceptions certainly abound regarding weight training. For example, most people think more is better—the heavier the weight, the more sets, and the more repetitions, the better the workout. Not true. If you do the exercises correctly, you can benefit from very little weight and relatively few repetitions, as the workout below will demonstrate.

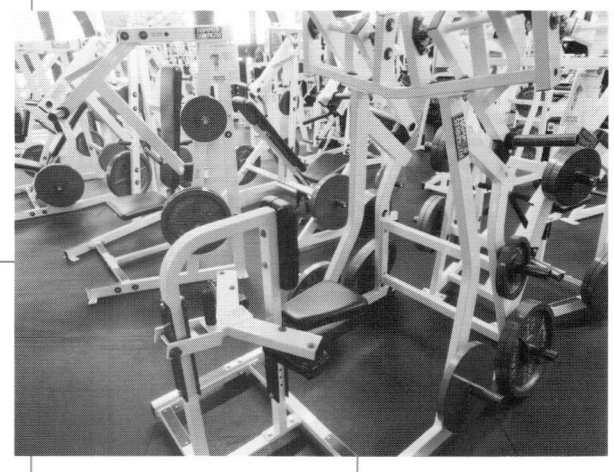

You may feel overwhelmed by all the different kinds of equipment in the gym. On first sight, the place can look like a medieval torture chamber. But in the descriptions later in this chapter, we'll show you which machines to start out on and exactly how to use them. The machines are excellent tools for beginners because when they're used correctly, they can help program your muscles to do the exercises correctly, within the proper range of motion, so that when you begin using free weights, you will be less likely to injure yourself.

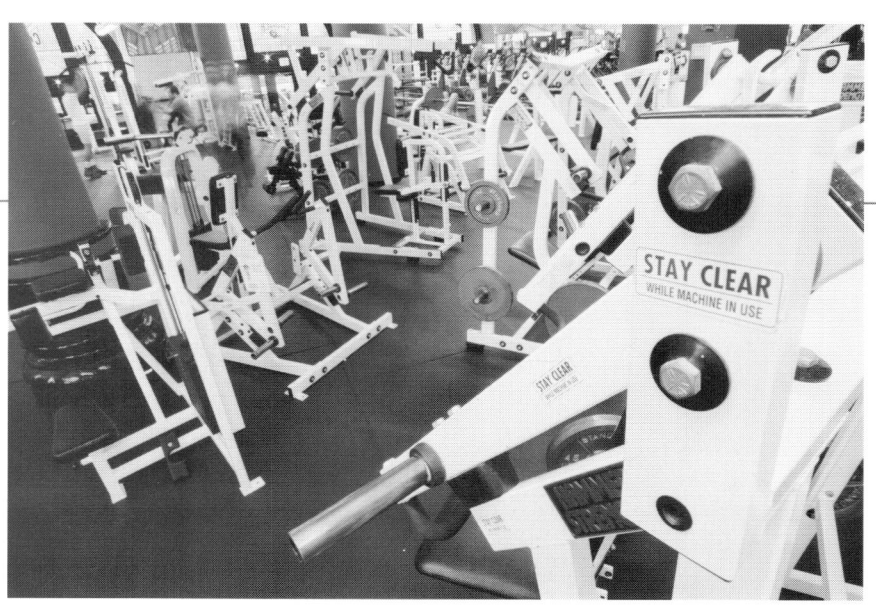

THE WORKOUT

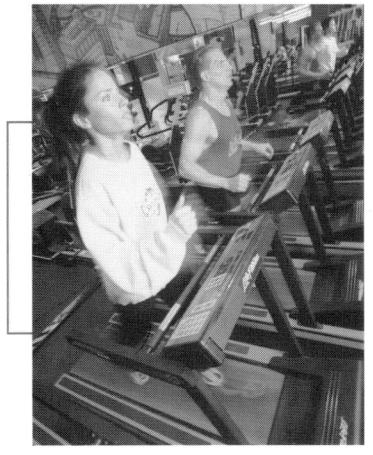

Cardio training. Cardiovascular training is the part of the workout that targets your most important muscle—your heart. Any sport or exercise that gets your heart rate up consistently over a period of time helps to improve your heart's efficiency. Cardio training is also called aerobic exercise—the term "aerobic" refers to the amount of oxygen that's being delivered to your muscles. As your heart efficiently pumps freshly oxygenated blood to your various muscles, you're increasing your "aerobic capacity."

The goal of cardio training is to sustain activity at your target heart rate, which is 60 to 75% of your maximum heart rate. Your maximum heart rate is determined by subtracting your age from 220. Let's use a 20-year old as an example:

220 minus 20 years = 200 beats per minute (bpm)

200 bpm = maximum heart rate

60 to 75% intensity = 120 to 150 beats per minute

Heart rate monitors offer the most convenient readings, but a more practical approach is a six-second pulse count. Count the number of beats you feel in six seconds and multiply that by 10. For example, if our 20-year old counts 14 beats in six seconds, she is exercising at 140 beats per minute—well within her target heart rate zone.

Regular cardio workouts at your target heart rate will lower your heart rate when you're at rest. That is a good thing because it means your heart does not have to work as hard to maintain circulation when you're not exercising (which is most of the time). Your heart becomes more efficient.

You have lots of options for cardio training—walking, jogging, biking, hiking, swimming, or playing tennis, racquetball, or another sport. As a beginner, your goal should be to try to exercise aerobically for 20 minutes at your target heart rate. As time goes on, you can work up to a full hour of cardio activity.

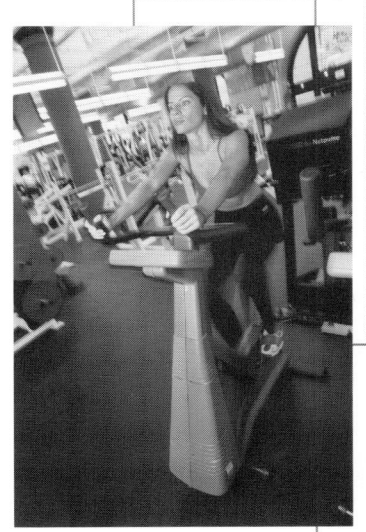

Flexibility training. Stretching is not just something you should do for 60 seconds before you go for a jog. Improving your flexibility is essential to avoid injury while you're doing the cardio and strength workouts. For that reason, stretching should be an integral part of every day's workout.

THE PROGRAM

Here are some options for scheduling your workouts. Choose the option that best fits your schedule.

Option 1
Day 1: Cardio: 20 to 30 minutes. Strength: Work all muscle groups.
Day 2: Rest
Day 3: Cardio and Strength Training
Day 4: Rest
Day 5: Cardio and Strength Training
Day 6: Cardio only.
Day 7: Rest

Option 2
Day 1: Cardio: 20 to 30 minutes. Strength: Work lower body muscle groups and abs.
Day 2: Cardio and upper body workout.
Day 3: Cardio only.
Day 4: Cardio and lower body and ab workout.
Day 5: Cardio and upper body workout.
Day 6: Cardio only (preferably outdoors).
Day 7: Rest

Option 3
Day 1: Cardio training: Start with 20 minutes of your favorite cardio activity, and over the course of several weeks, work up to 45 minutes.
Day 2: Strength training: Work all muscle groups on each day of strength training.
Day 3: Cardio training
Day 4: Strength training
Day 5: Cardio training
Day 6: Strength training
Day 7: Rest

THE WORKOUT

Never do strength training two days in a row! Your muscles need time to repair, and if you don't give them enough time, you *will* injure yourself. Working out with weights causes micro traumas to the muscles. Repairing these micro traumas actually makes the muscle leaner and stronger. If you don't allow enough time for the muscles to

TRAIN AROUND INJURIES

When ball players injure their shoulders or hamstrings or knees, do they fly down to the Bahamas and sit on the beach for a month? No, they keep training *around* their injuries so that the rest of their muscles that aren't hurt stay toned. Professionals in sports medicine help them keep the rest of their bodies in shape so that they can get back on the playing field as soon as possible.

If you suffer an injury, consider training around it so that you can get back on the playing field of your life as soon as possible. Your doctor may send you to physical therapy, but those exercises are meant to rehabilitate just the injured area. Ask your doctor if it's safe to exercise the rest of your body while your injury is healing. Don't use an injury as an excuse to abandon your overall physical fitness!

repair themselves, however, these micro traumas will develop into macro traumas (i.e., injuries)!

There are no exceptions to this rule. Some people believe that the abdominal muscles are the exception and that they can do crunches or other ab exercises every day. Not true! You may want that flat stomach more than you want, say, a nicely toned bicep, but wanting something more doesn't mean you should exercise it more!

THE WARM-UP

Most people think of a warm-up as a few stretches. Don't be one of those people! You do not want to stretch cold muscles. Think of your muscles as a rubber band that's been in the freezer. If you bend it, it's going to snap. Your muscles are no different. A warm-up should always be done *before* stretching!

So what's a good warm-up? About five to 10 minutes of light cardiovascular exercise—jogging, jumping rope, doing jumping jacks, etc. This activity not only brings some warm blood to the muscles, but it also releases *synovial fluid*, which is a sort of joint lubricant. By lubricating the joints and muscles, this fluid helps prevent a lot of common joint injuries.

BEGINNER'S LUCK

GYM ETIQUETTE

The most muscle-bound weight lifter who doesn't know his salad fork from his butter knife knows basic gym etiquette. Unfortunately, beginners who don't have fitness pros to help guide them are often confronted with a subculture that's completely foreign to them. Here are some basic courtesies you should know about:

First, always towel off the machine you've been using when you're done. No one likes to sit down on a wet bench!

Second, replace weights when you're done with them.

Third, learn to share equipment. How exactly? Well, you'll notice some gym members may ask you, when you're in the middle of a set, if they can "work in" on your machine. This does not mean that they are asking you to leave. They also are not asking you how many sets you have left. They want to know if you will let them do one set when you are done with your current set, then they'll let you continue with your next set, and so on. Do *not* say, "I just have two more sets to do!" Remember, you need to rest between sets, and the time it takes the other person to do his or her set is the time your muscles need to rest.

When you start working in, you'll notice that the gym, which may seem at first like a completely unstructured, chaotic place, actually has a flow to it.

FLEXIBILITY TRAINING

After the warm-up, you're ready to stretch. If you're doing cardiovascular training for your day's workout, you can do the full-body stretch described below. On weight training days, we've incorporated the stretches right into the workout (which is described later).

Don't worry if you can't complete each stretch your first time trying—just stretch as far as you can. You will gradually improve your flexibility as time goes on.

Hold each position for 15 seconds unless otherwise noted.

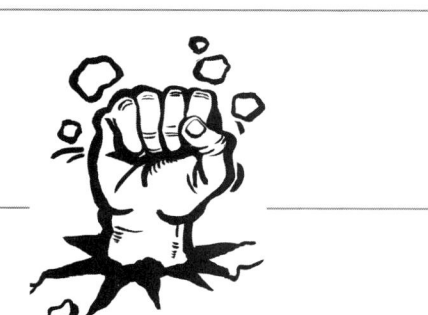

THE WORKOUT

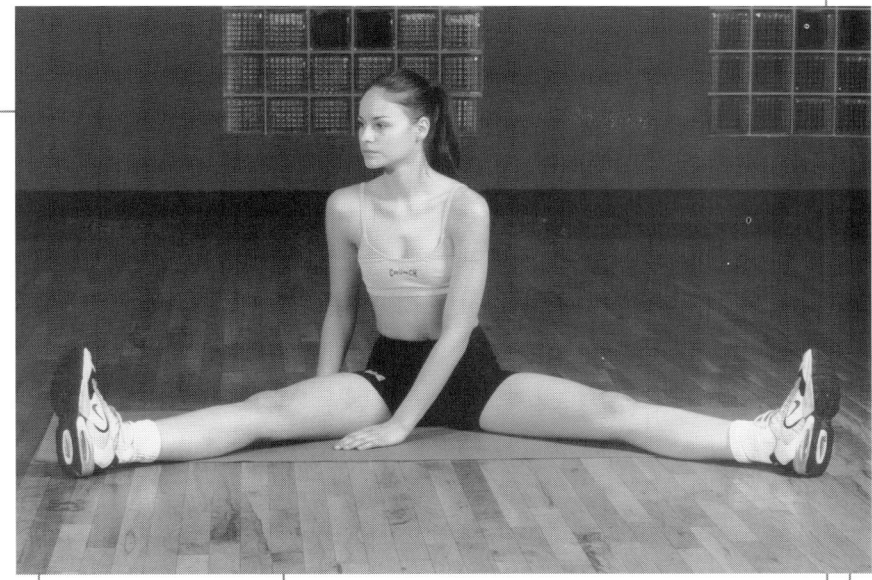

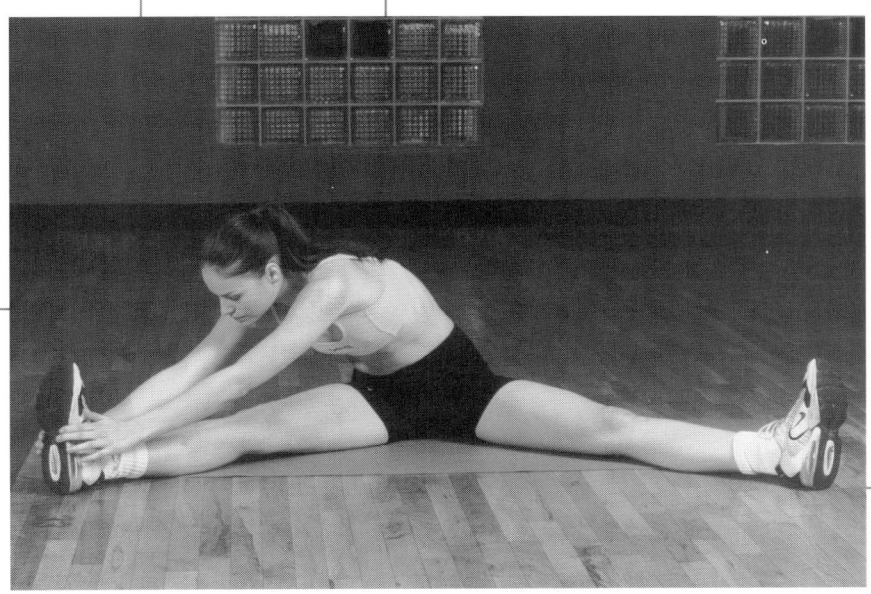

Sitting with legs straight out in a wide straddle, reach down your right side, bringing chest as close to knee as you can. You don't have to be able to touch your feet. Repeat on left side.

BEGINNER'S LUCK

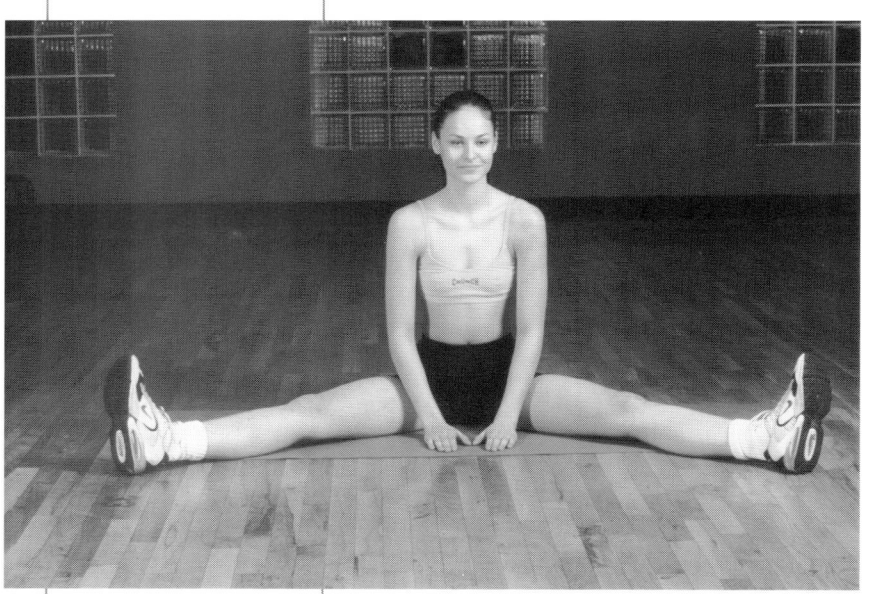

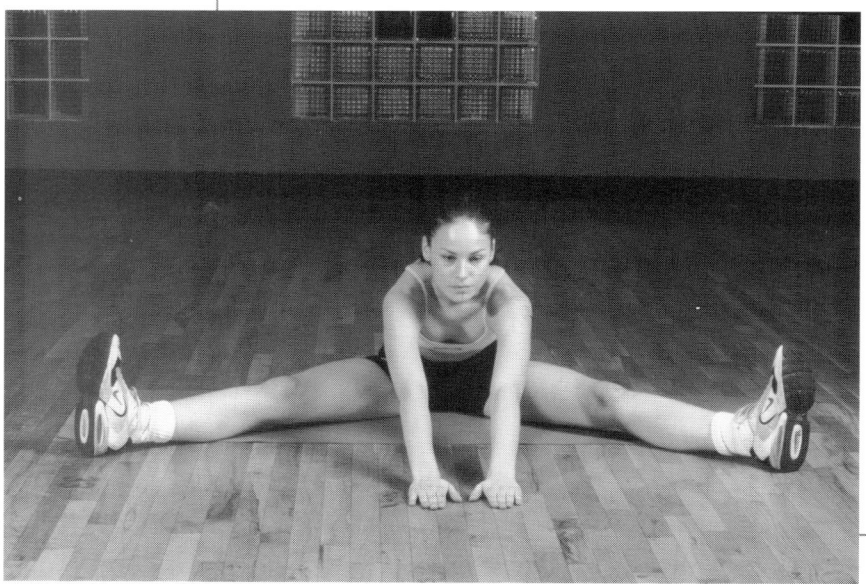

Walk hands up the middle, bringing chest as close to floor between your legs as you can.

THE WORKOUT

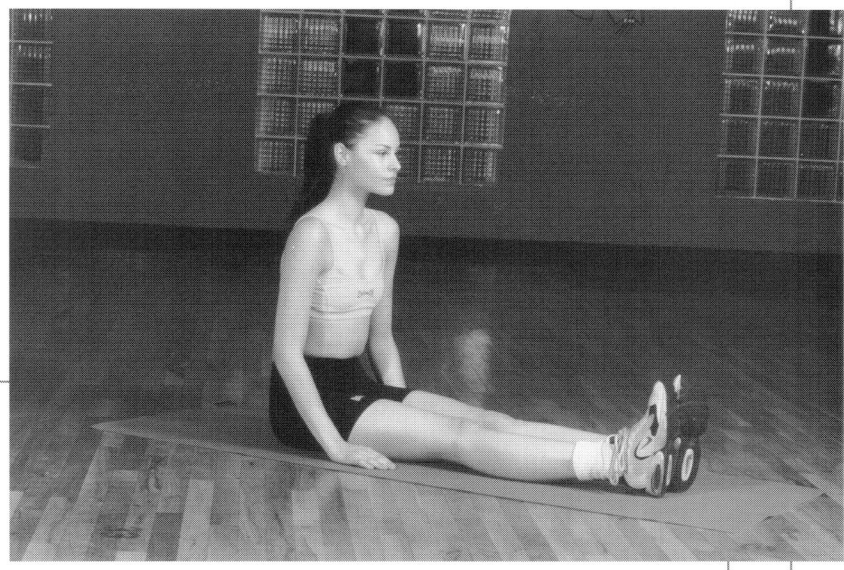

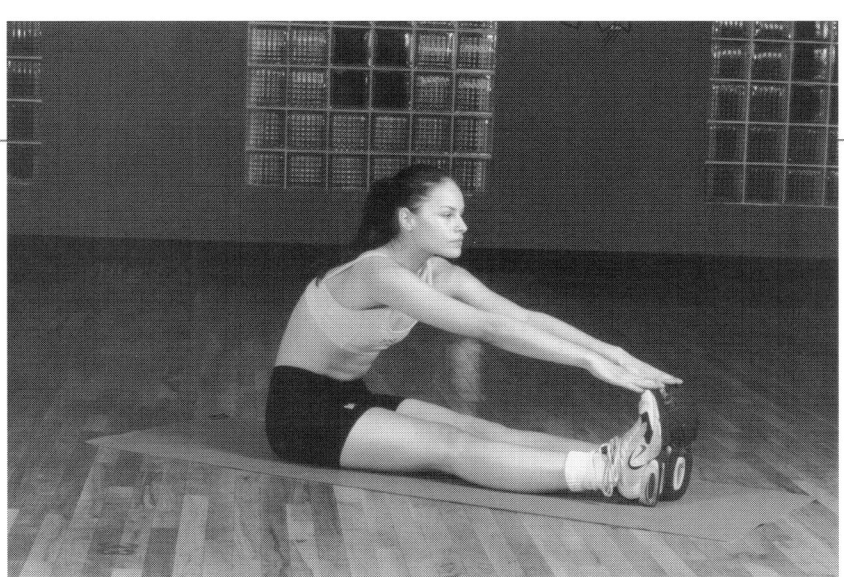

Bring legs together and walk your hands up toward your feet. This is a pike stretch.

BEGINNER'S LUCK

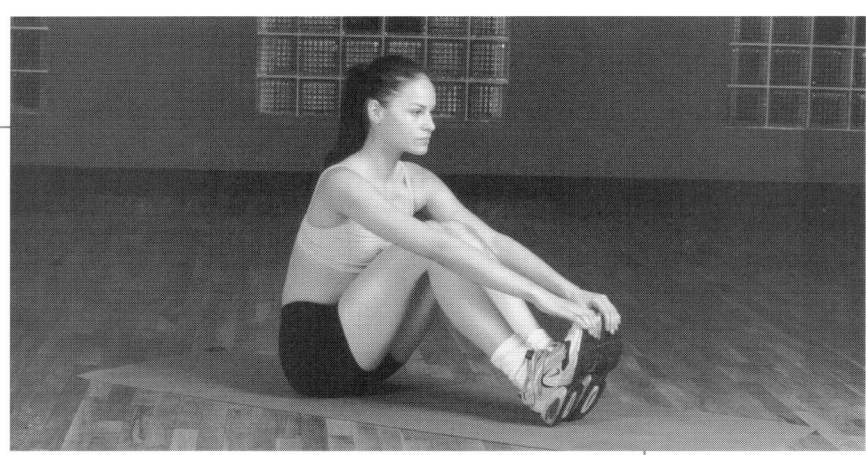

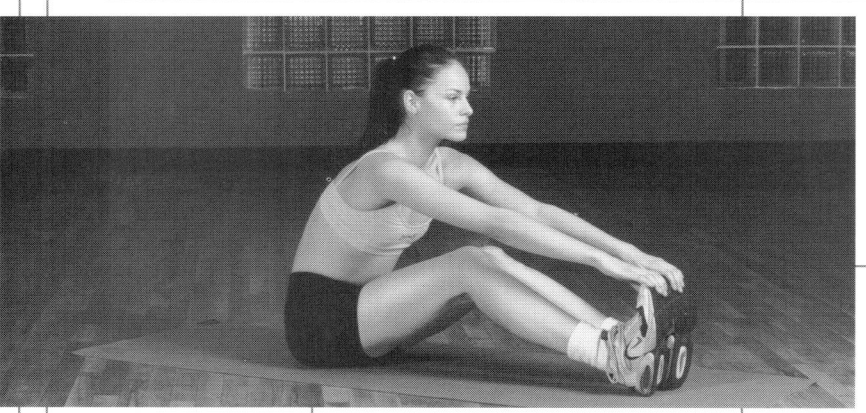

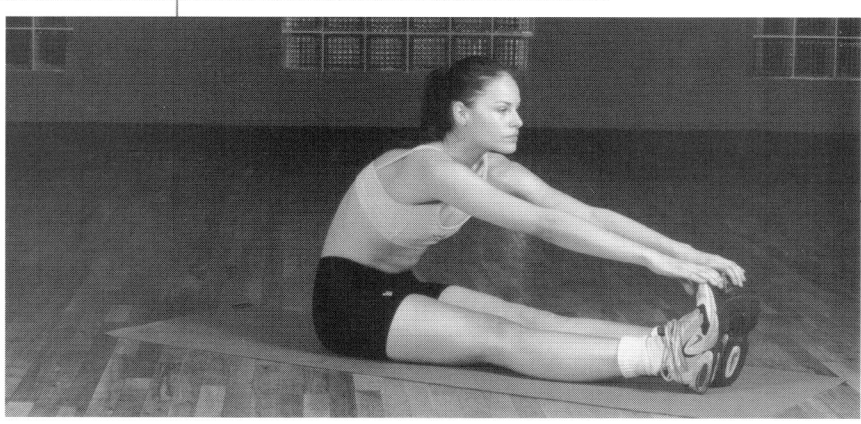

Bring knees up to chest and grab your toes. Straighten legs out as much as you can. Flex your toes and pull back.

THE WORKOUT

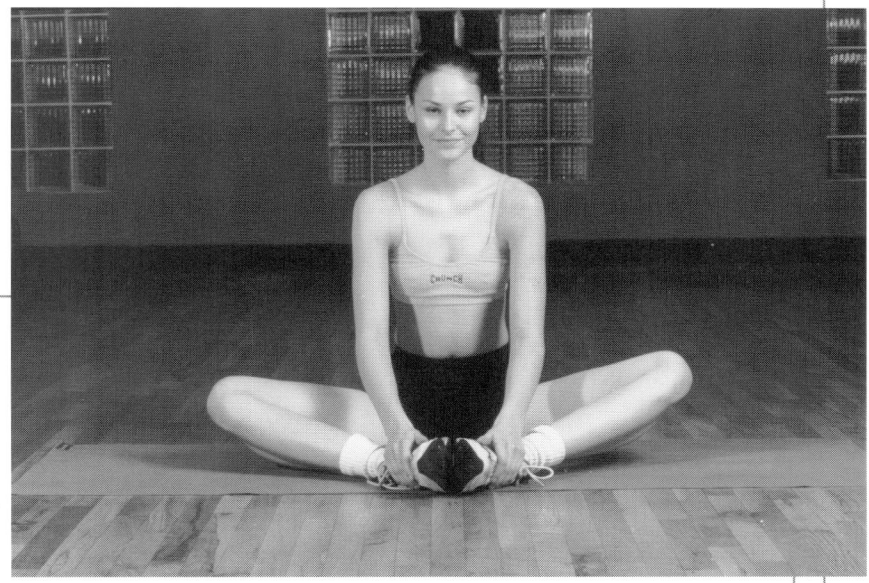

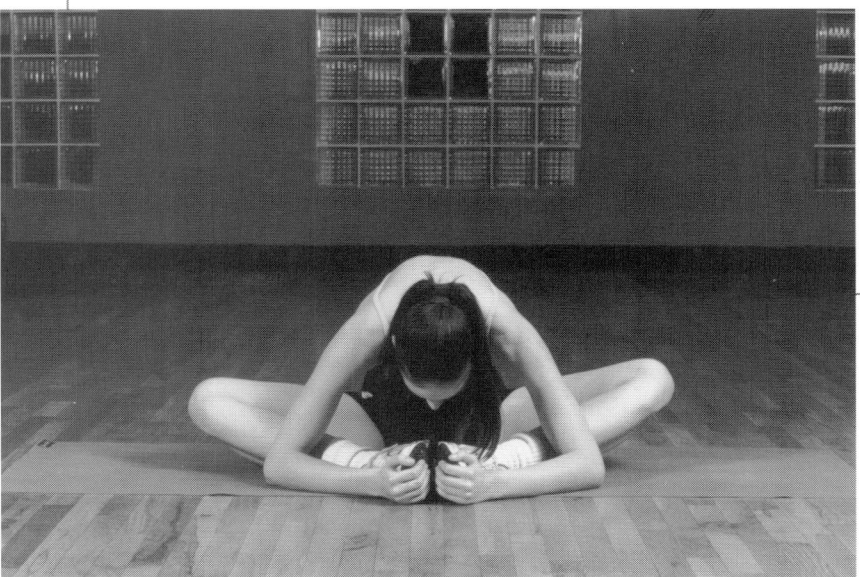

Bring your feet into your middle in a butterfly position. Put your hands on your feet and put your head down.

BEGINNER'S LUCK

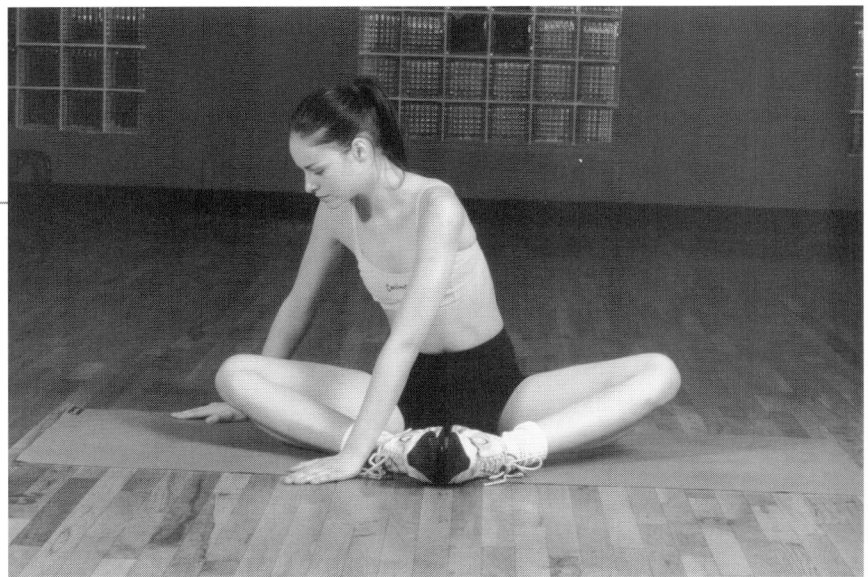

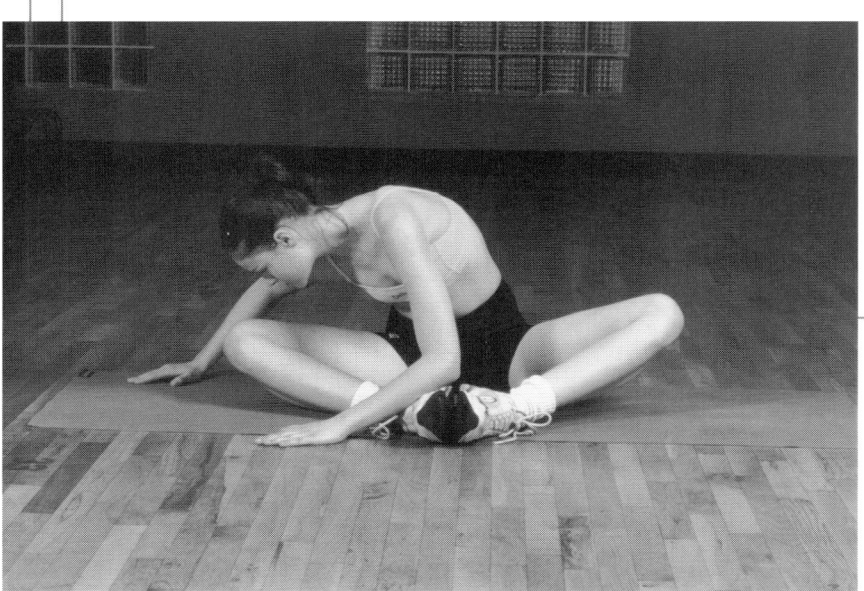

Placing your hands on the floor on either side of your knee, lower your head toward your knee. Repeat on other side.

THE WORKOUT

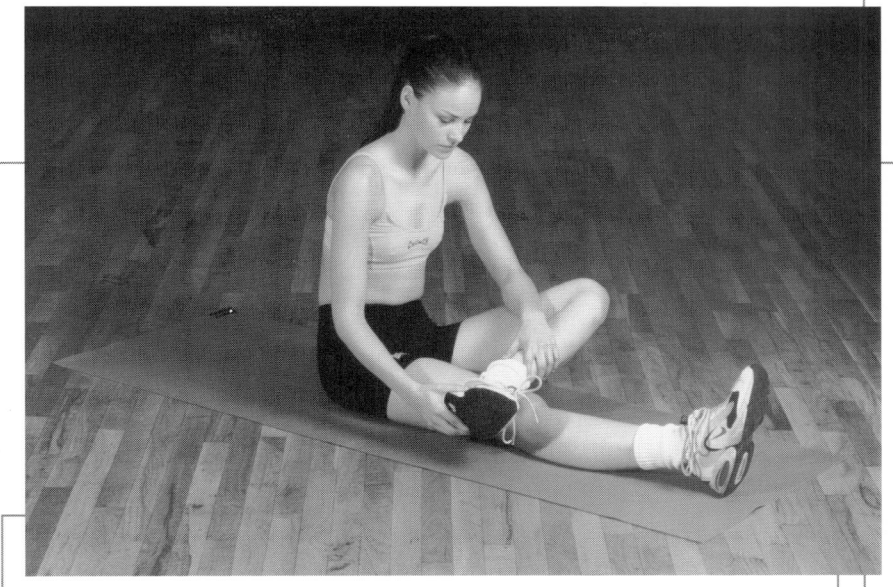

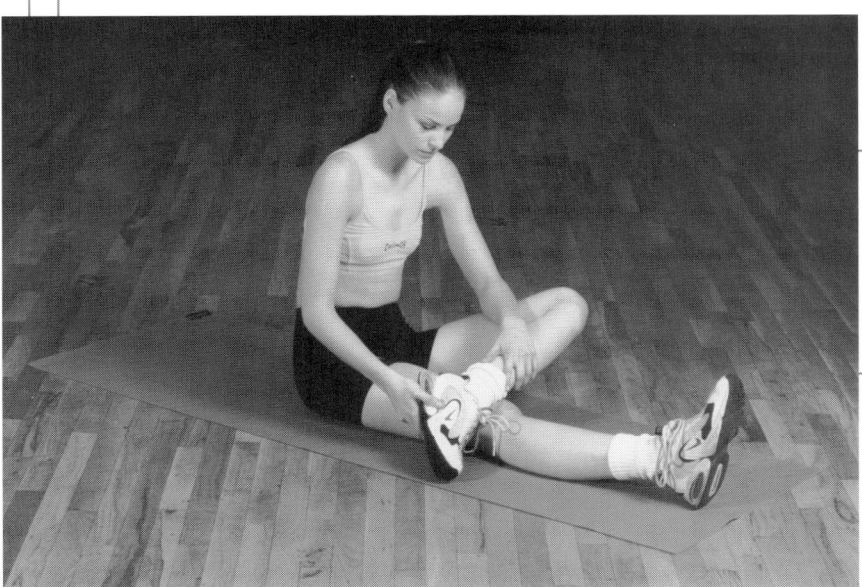

Put one leg out straight and put opposite leg's foot to straight leg's knee. Rotate ankle each way.

BEGINNER'S LUCK

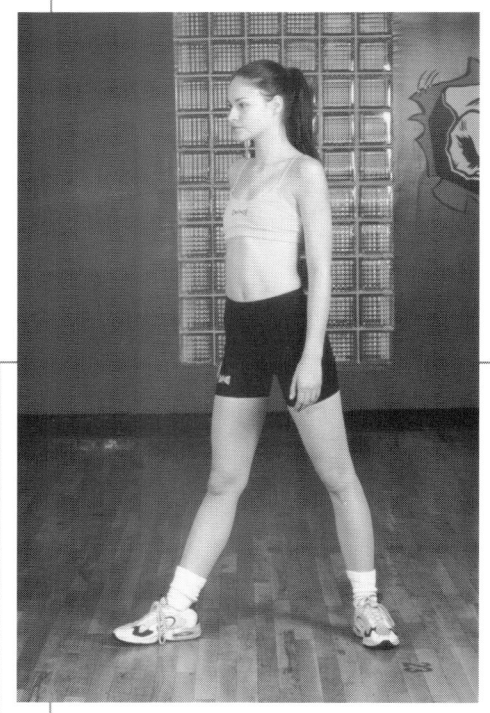
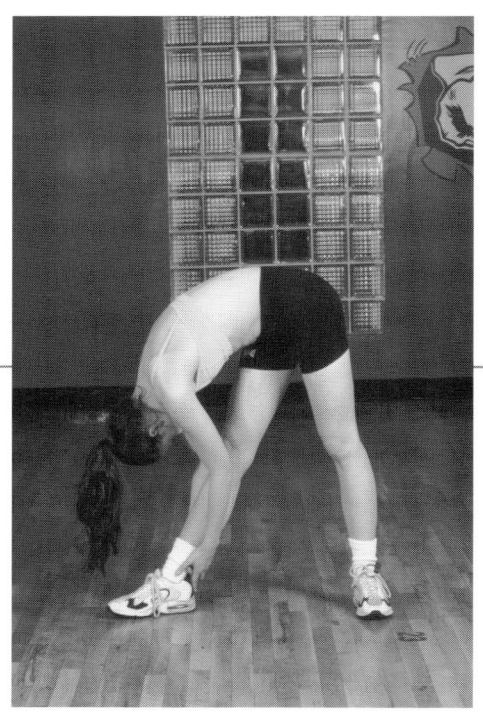

Stand up, with legs apart and feet pointing out. Turn body to the right, making sure your chest is in line with your knee. Work hands down your right side to your feet. Repeat on left side.

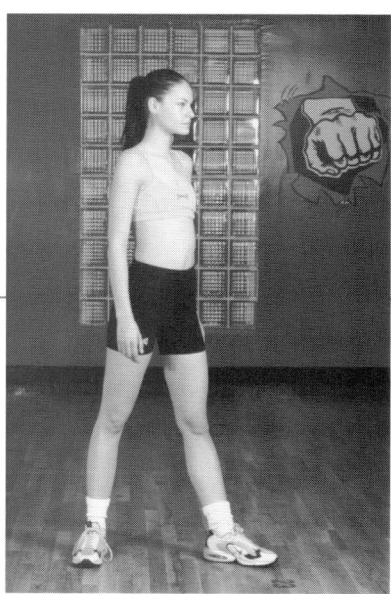
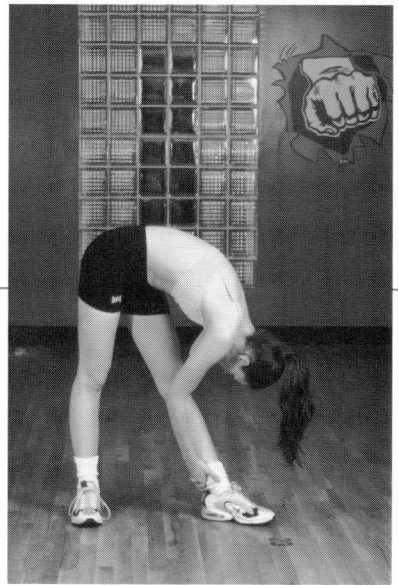

THE WORKOUT

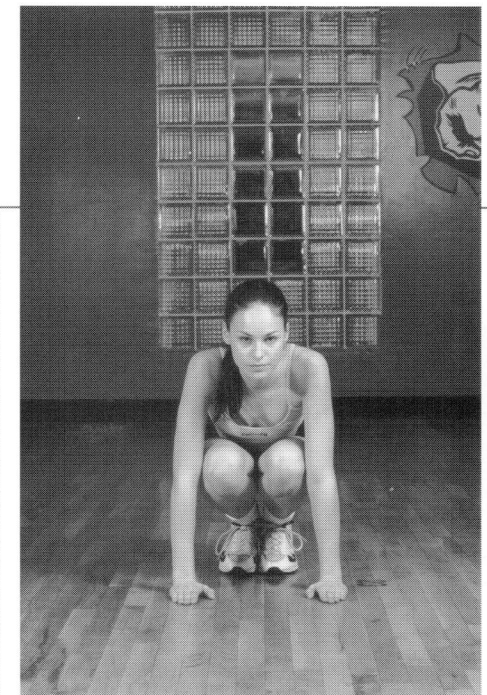

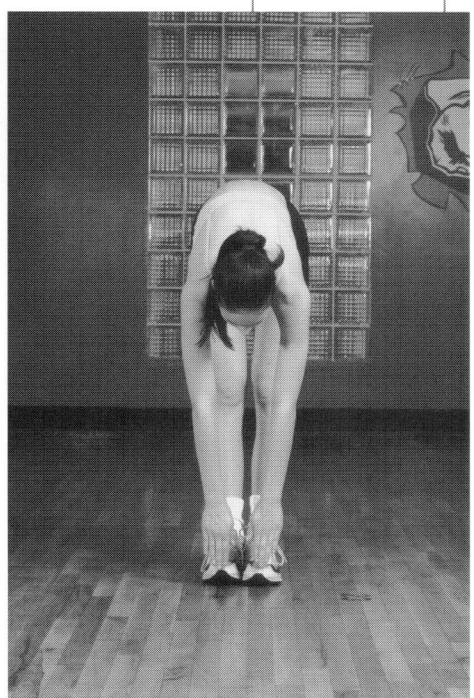

Squat with knees together and place hands on the floor in front of you. Lift your butt up while grasping your toes.

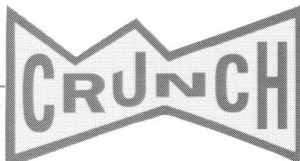

BEGINNER'S LUCK

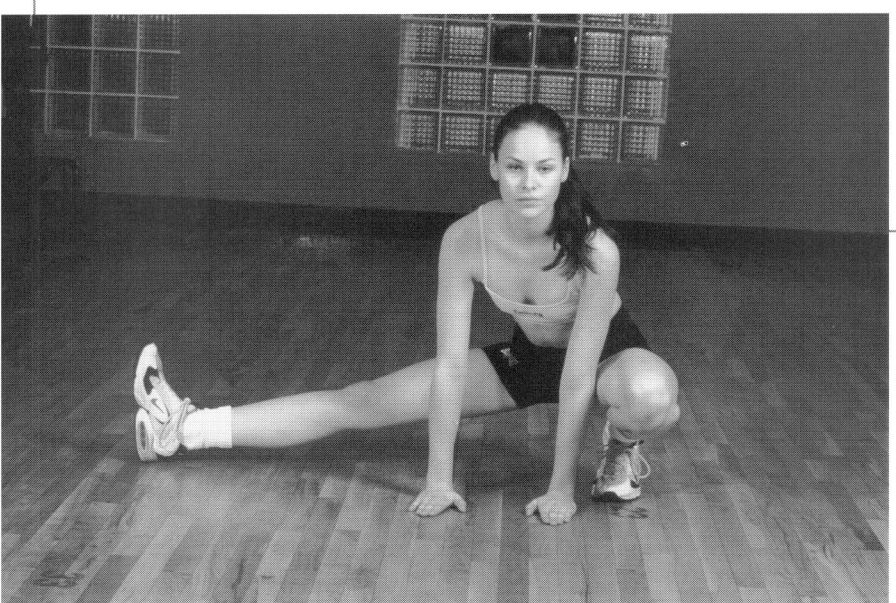

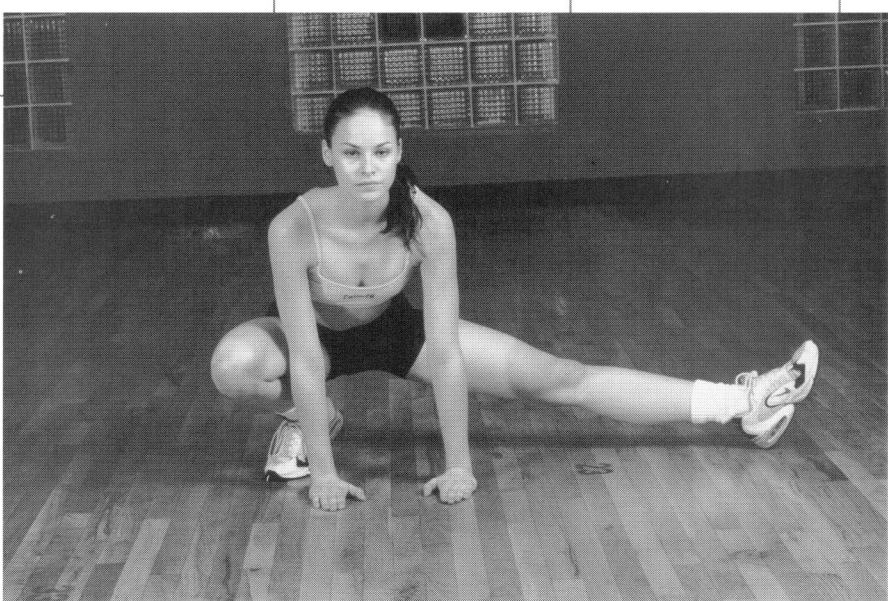

Standing with legs together, squat down. Fully extend right leg, putting hands flat on the floor. Your right heel should touch the ground. Don't hyperextend your knee. Hold for 10 seconds. Repeat on opposite side. Do two sets.

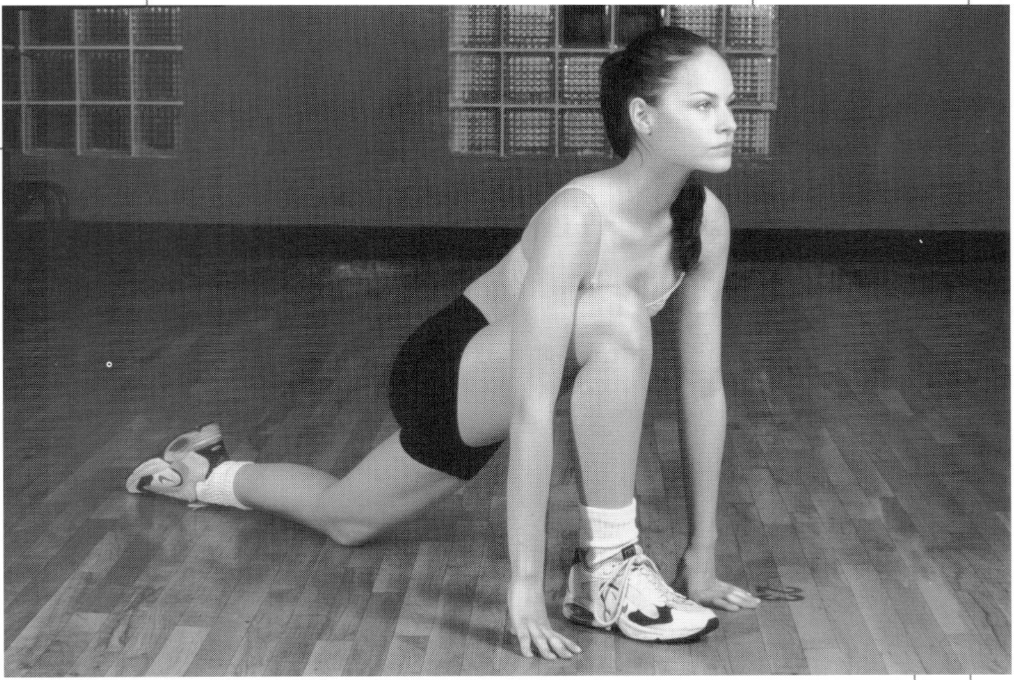

THE WORKOUT

Lunge, putting one knee to the floor. Keep hips square. Put hands down and stretch forward, bringing chest down. Turn heel out. Repeat with opposite leg.

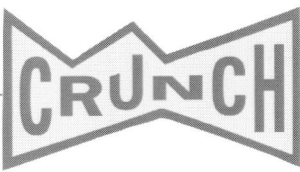

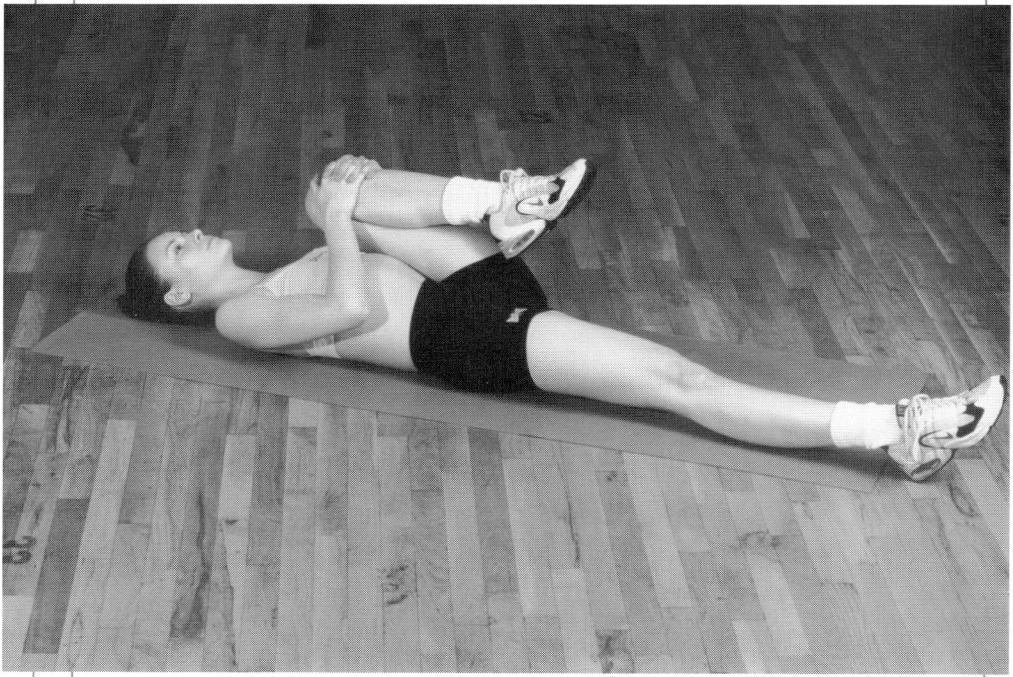

BEGINNER'S LUCK

Lie on your back. Pull one leg up in to your chest. Repeat with other leg.

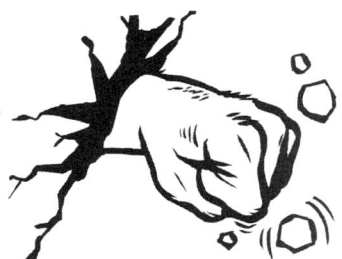

THE WORKOUT

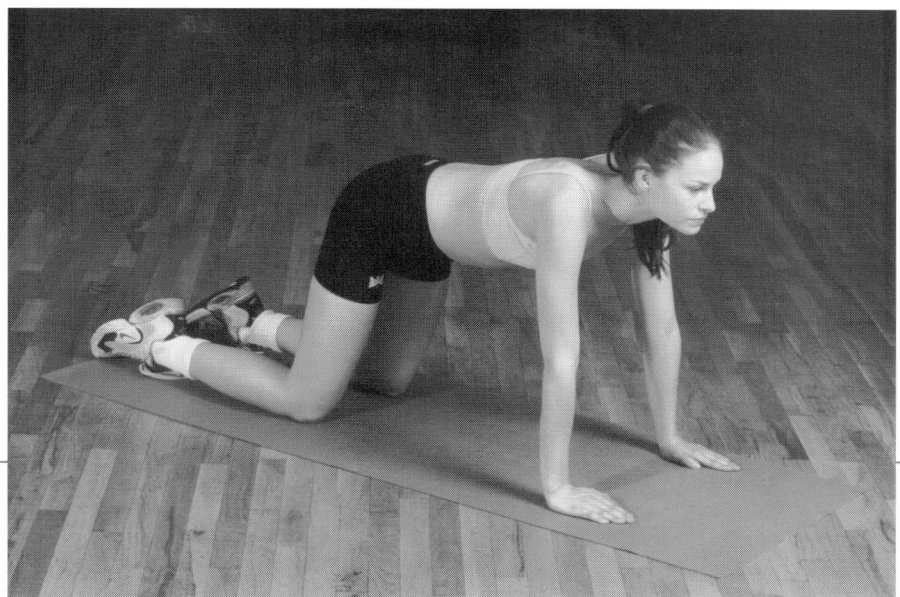

On all fours, bring your head down to the ground and stretch your arms stretched out. This is a cat stretch.

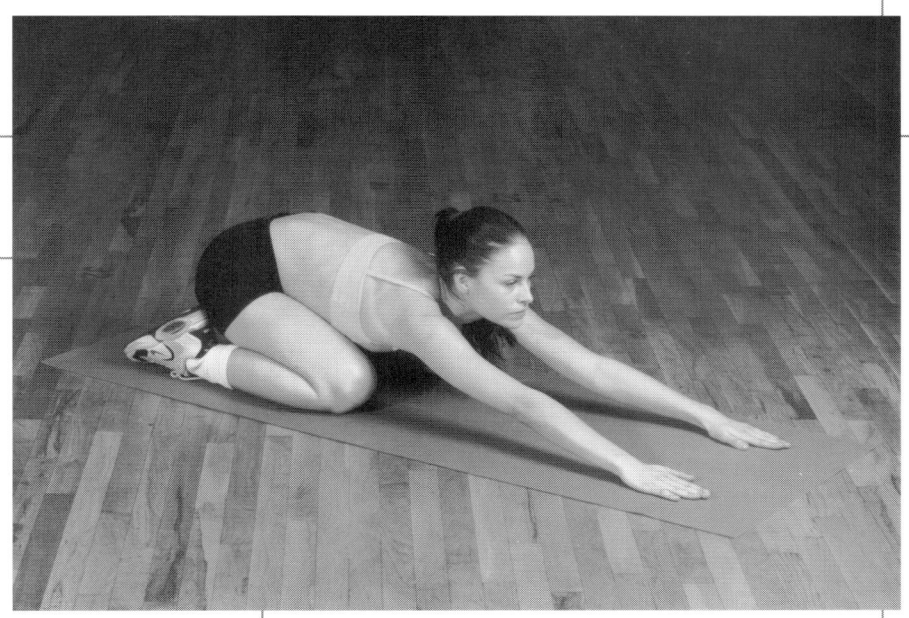

BEGINNER'S LUCK

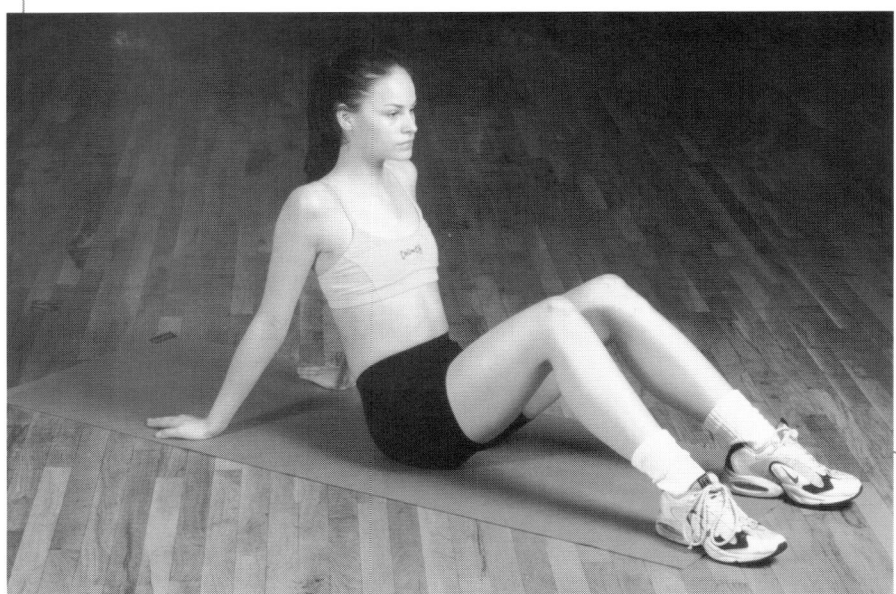

Flip over. With arms shoulder-length apart, hands on the floor with fingers pointing back, lift shoulders off ground and raise knees, keeping feet on floor. Keep your chest up. This is an M stretch.

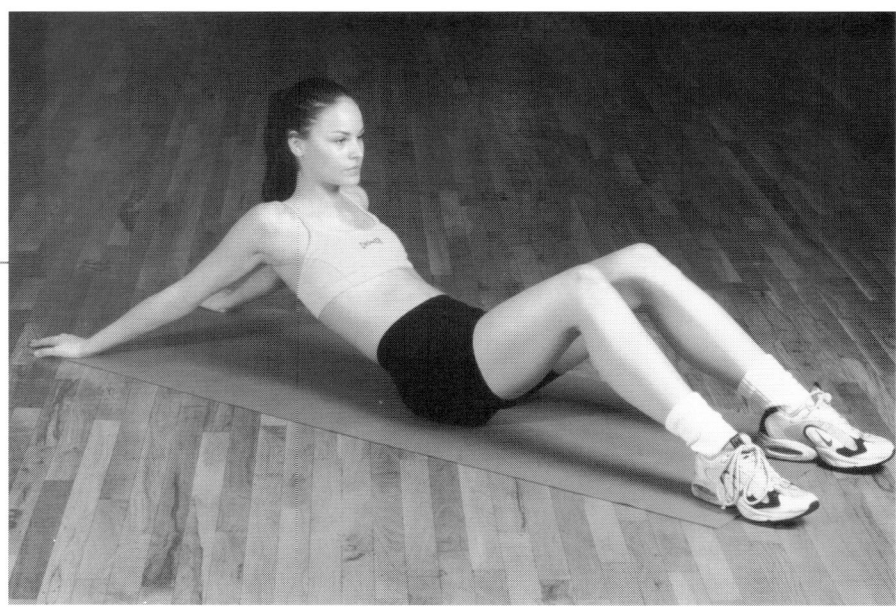

THE WORKOUT

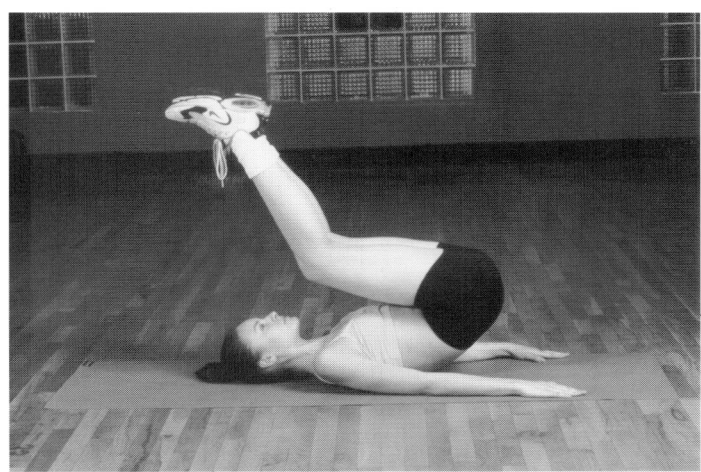

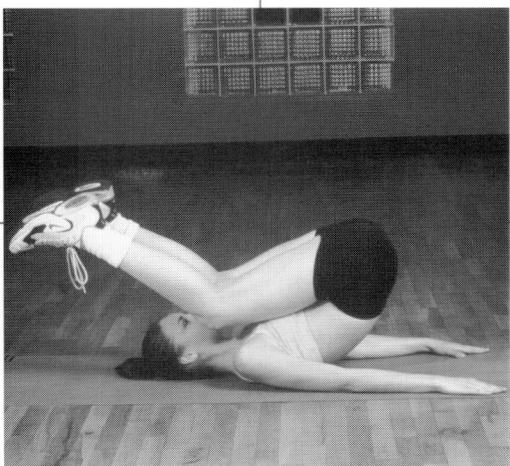
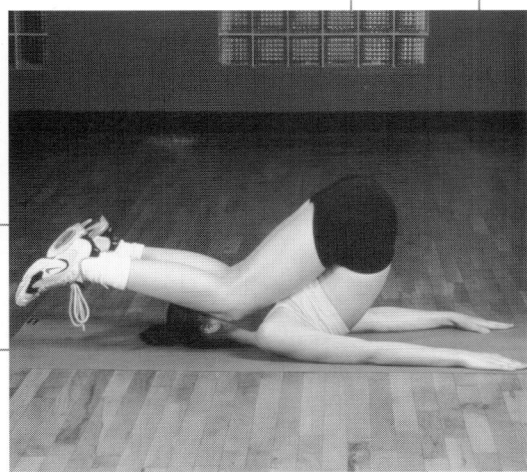

Lie down flat on your back. Kick legs over your head. Straddle your head, touch knees to the ground. Slowly roll legs back to the ground. Do twice.

BEGINNER'S LUCK

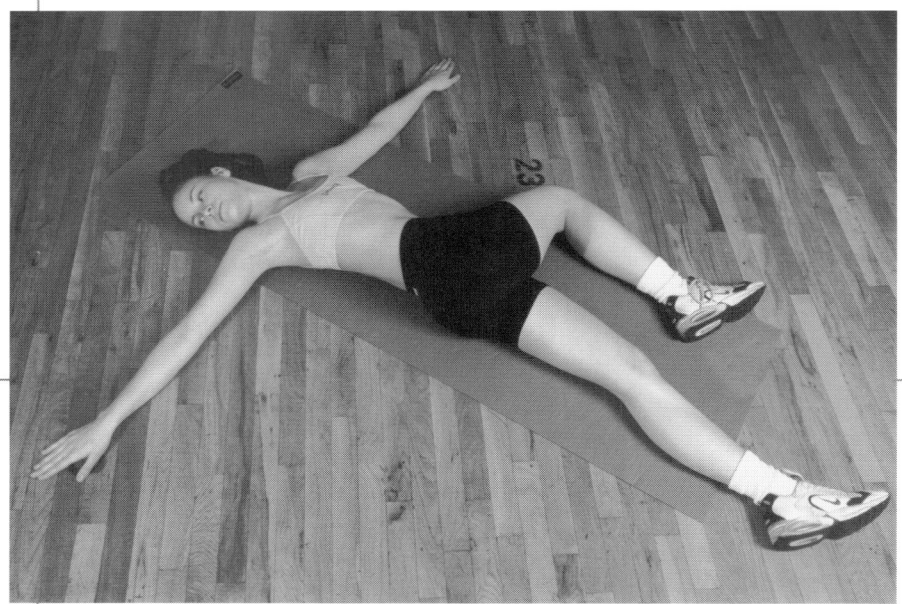

Lie flat on your back, with arms straight out to sides. Cross one leg over the other and turn head to look at opposite arm. Alternate sides. This is a good glute stretch. For a deeper stretch, change the height of the knee.

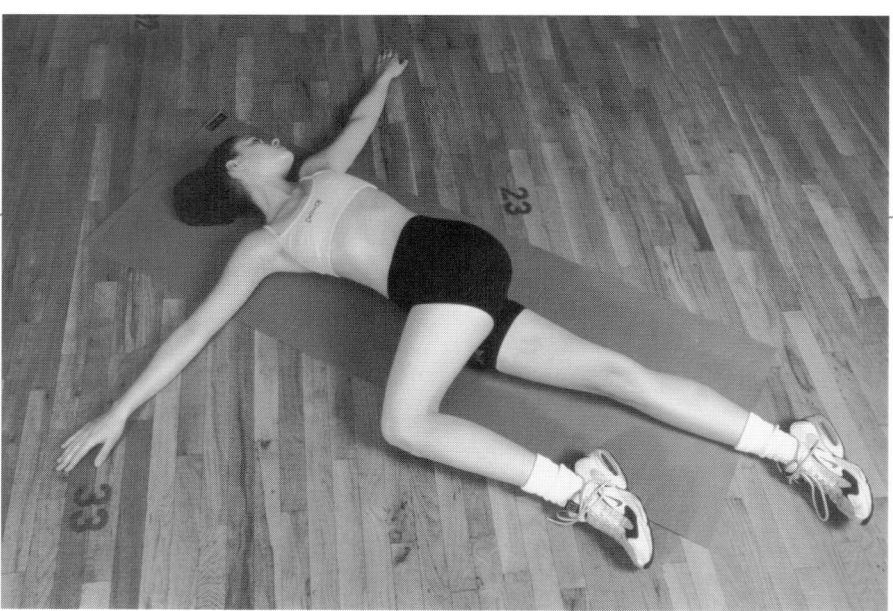

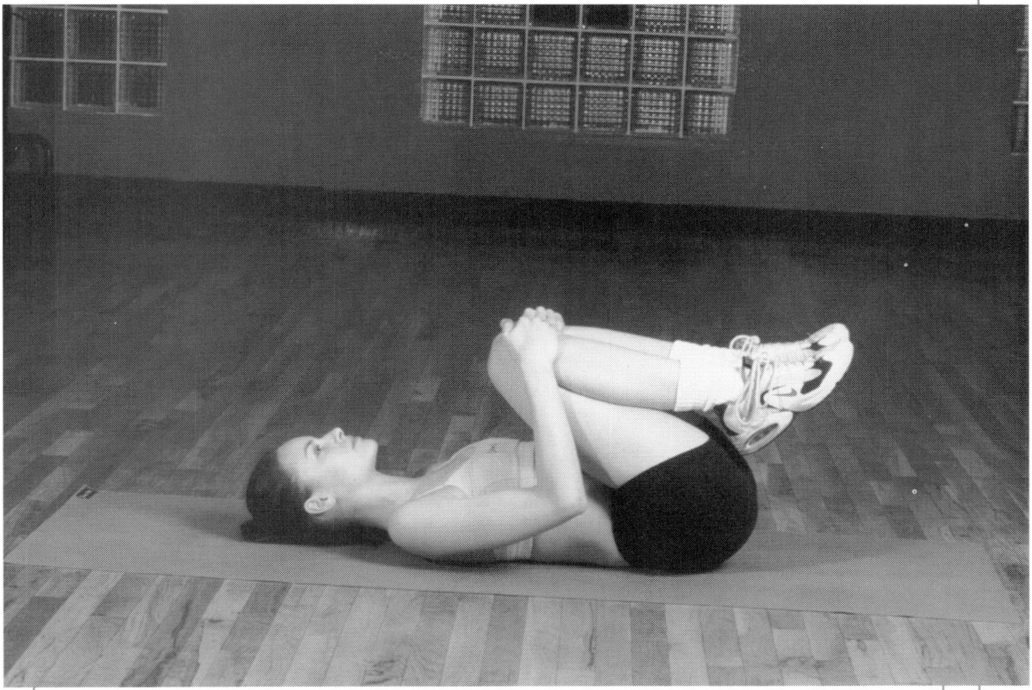

THE WORKOUT

Lie on your back, grab your knees and pull them up to your chest.

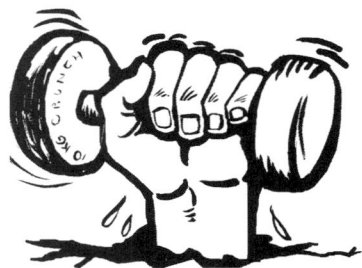

39

BEGINNER'S LUCK

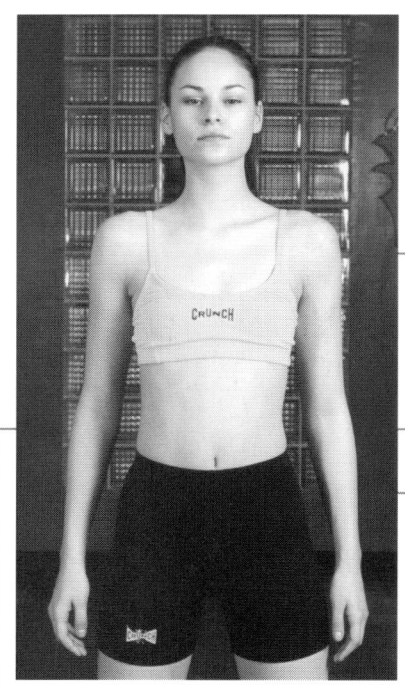
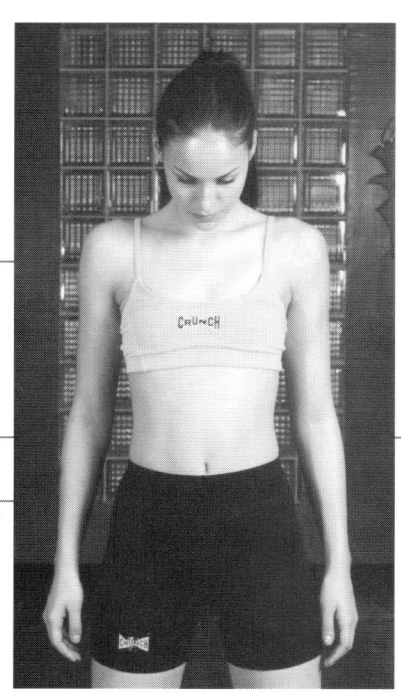

Do neck circles, but do not grind your neck *back*—it may damage your cartilage.

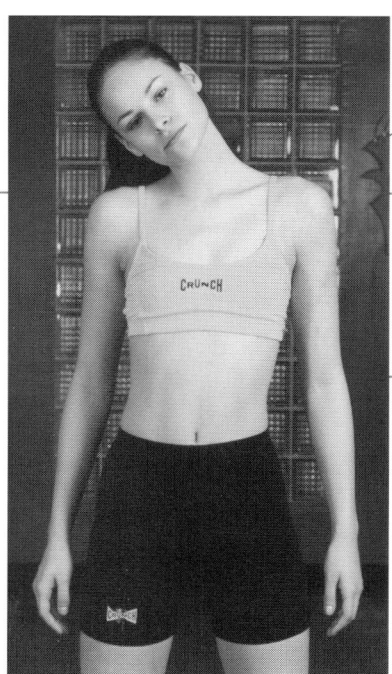
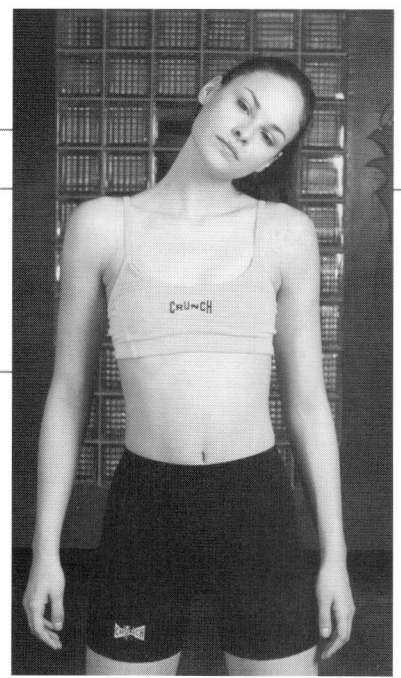

THE WORKOUT

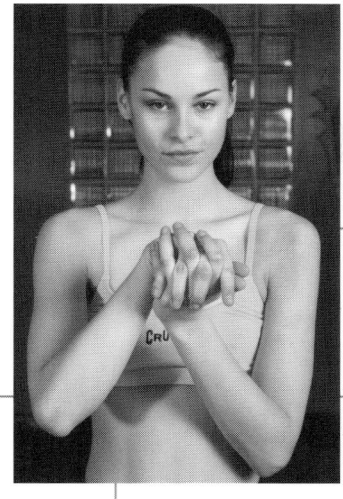
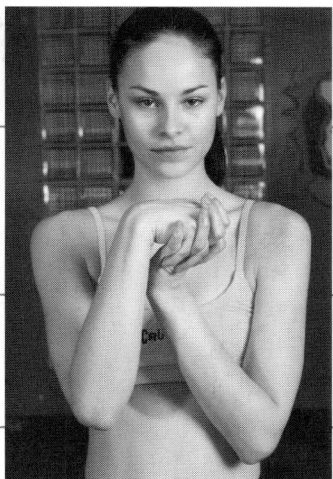

Clasp your hands together and rotate your wrist in circles.

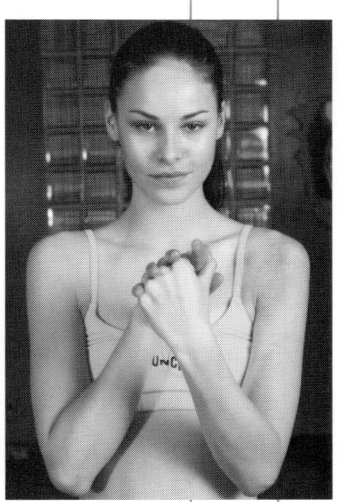
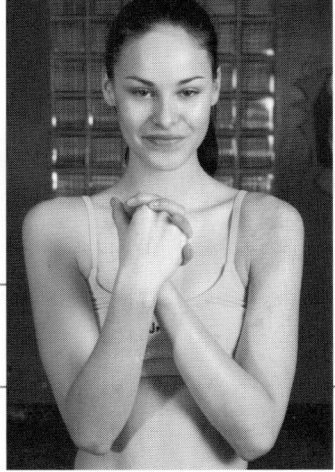
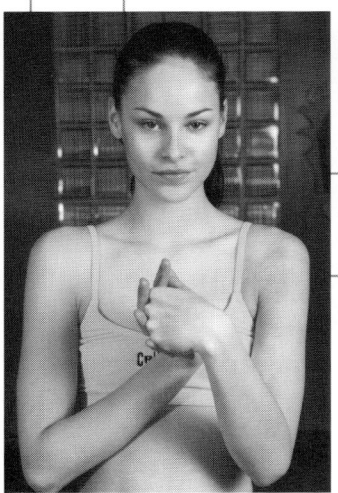

BEGINNER'S LUCK

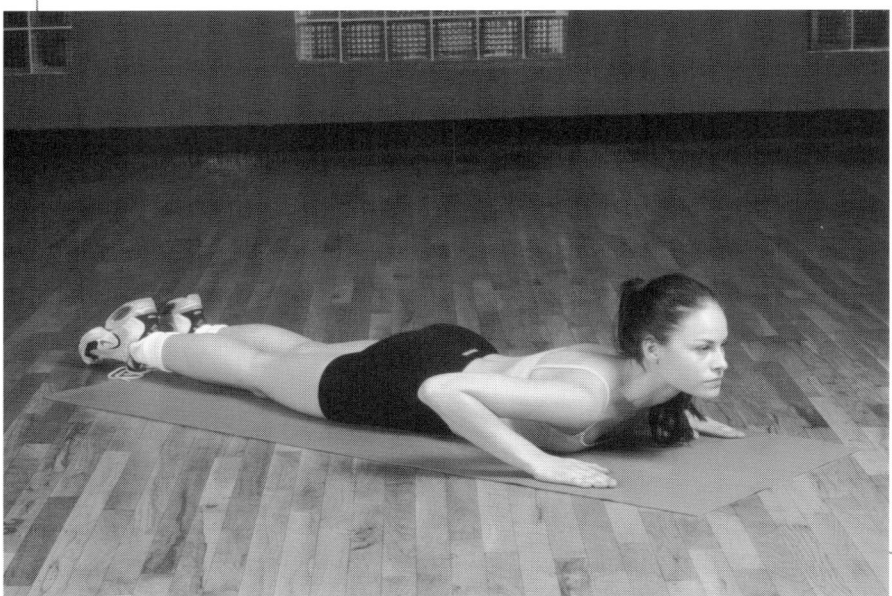

Lie on your stomach in the push-up position, and slowly push your chest up. Keep your hips on the ground and your neck back. This is a seal stretch.

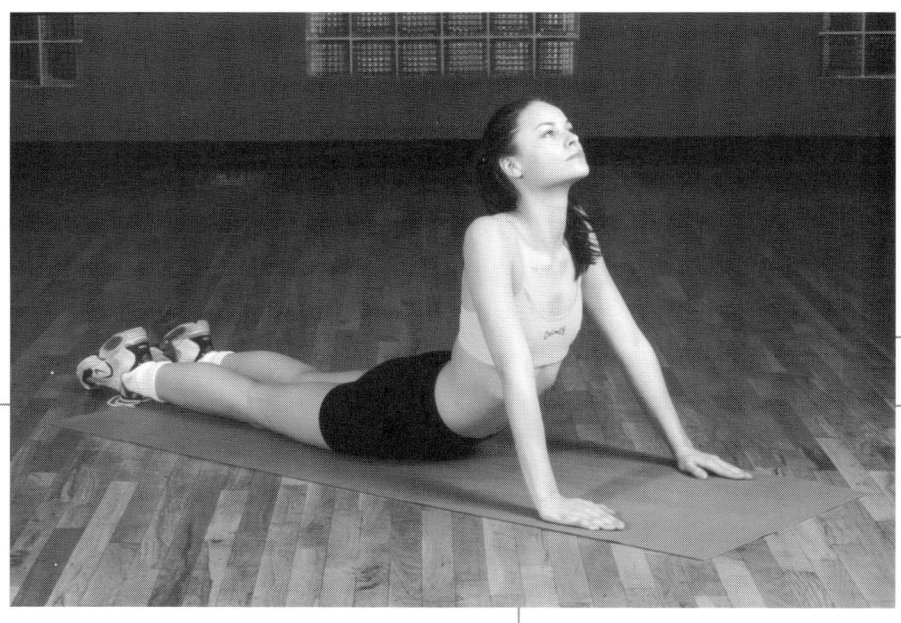

THE WORKOUT

STRENGTH TRAINING BASICS

Before you pick up a dumbbell and start doing reps, it helps to understand exactly what muscles you should be working and in what order. So let's take a look at what you're working with.

When strength training, you want to work your biggest muscle group first to avoid injury and get the most benefit from each exercise. Within each muscle group, you want to work the muscles in order of size, from biggest to smallest. That's because when you work the anatomically larger muscles, the anatomically smaller muscles assist them. If you work your smaller muscles first, they will be too fatigued to assist the larger ones when you then work the large muscles. Working your muscles in the proper order helps to prevent injuries to your muscles and your joints.

This workout is done in a "push/pull" order. Alternating exercises that work the "pull" muscles (extensors) with those that work the "push" muscles (flexors) allows the opposite muscles to rest during the workout.

With all this in mind, here is a list of the order in which you should work out your muscles:

1. Legs (otherwise known as quadriceps and hamstrings)
2. Hips (hip flexors)
3. Butt (glutes)
4. Chest (pectorals)
5. Back (latissimus dorsi, rhomboids, erector spinae)
6. Shoulders (deltoids, trapezius)
7. Biceps
8. Triceps
9. Abdominals (rectus abdominis, obliques)

The good news is that some exercises work more than one muscle, so you don't need to do separate exercises for each muscle. For example, squats work your glutes, hips, and quads, so there's no need to do separate "butt blasters" to tighten your tush.

You'll notice that obliques, the muscles that run down the sides of your torso, are missing from the list. Crunches and other abdominal exercises work the obliques to a good extent. Exercises specifically designed for obliques, such as side bends and pole twists, can injure your back. (What's more, if you work your obliques too much, they will get bigger—and a bigger middle is not most people's goal . . .)

The 12 basic exercises are as follows:

BEGINNER'S LUCK

MEET YOUR MUSCLES (BACK)

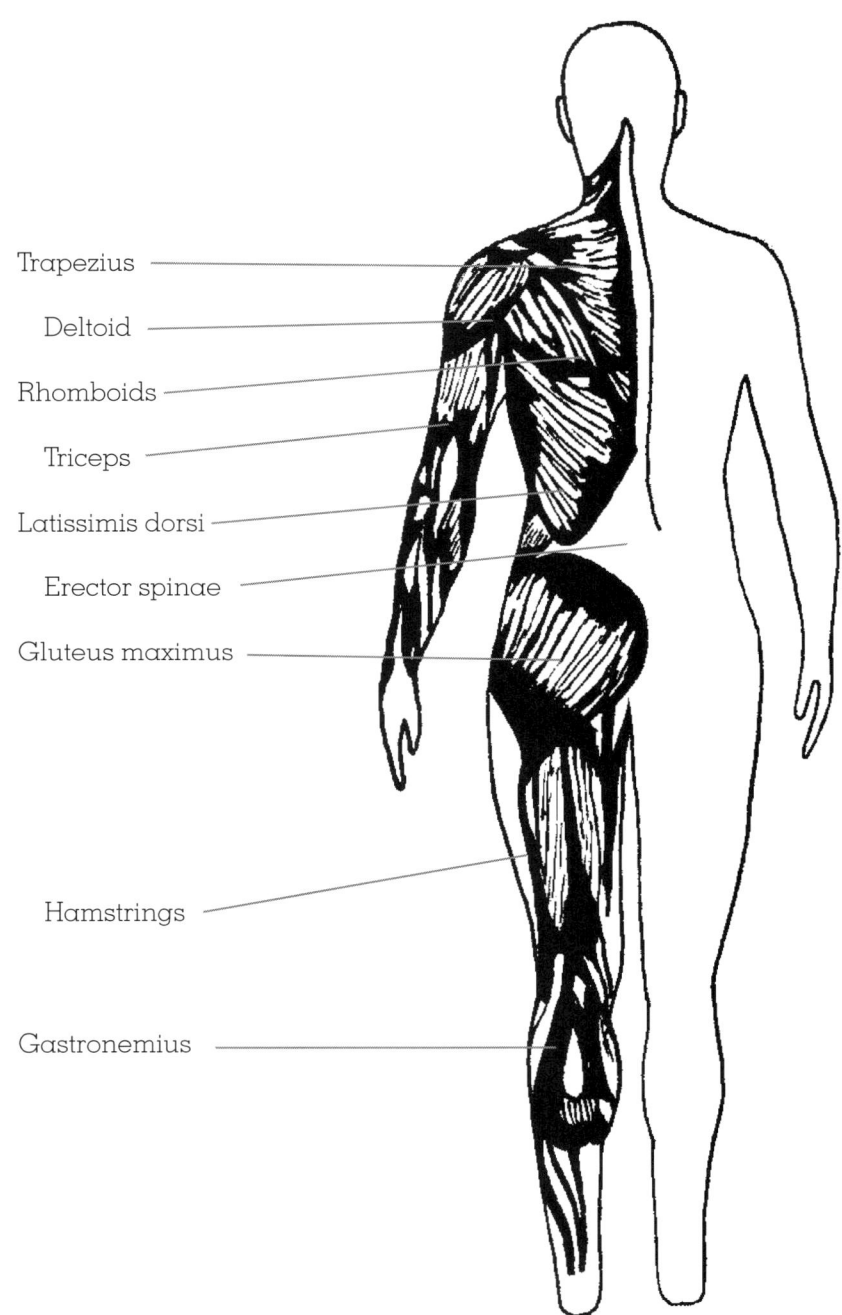

- Trapezius
- Deltoid
- Rhomboids
- Triceps
- Latissimis dorsi
- Erector spinae
- Gluteus maximus
- Hamstrings
- Gastronemius

"Meet Your Muscles" illustrations by Judi Ketchum

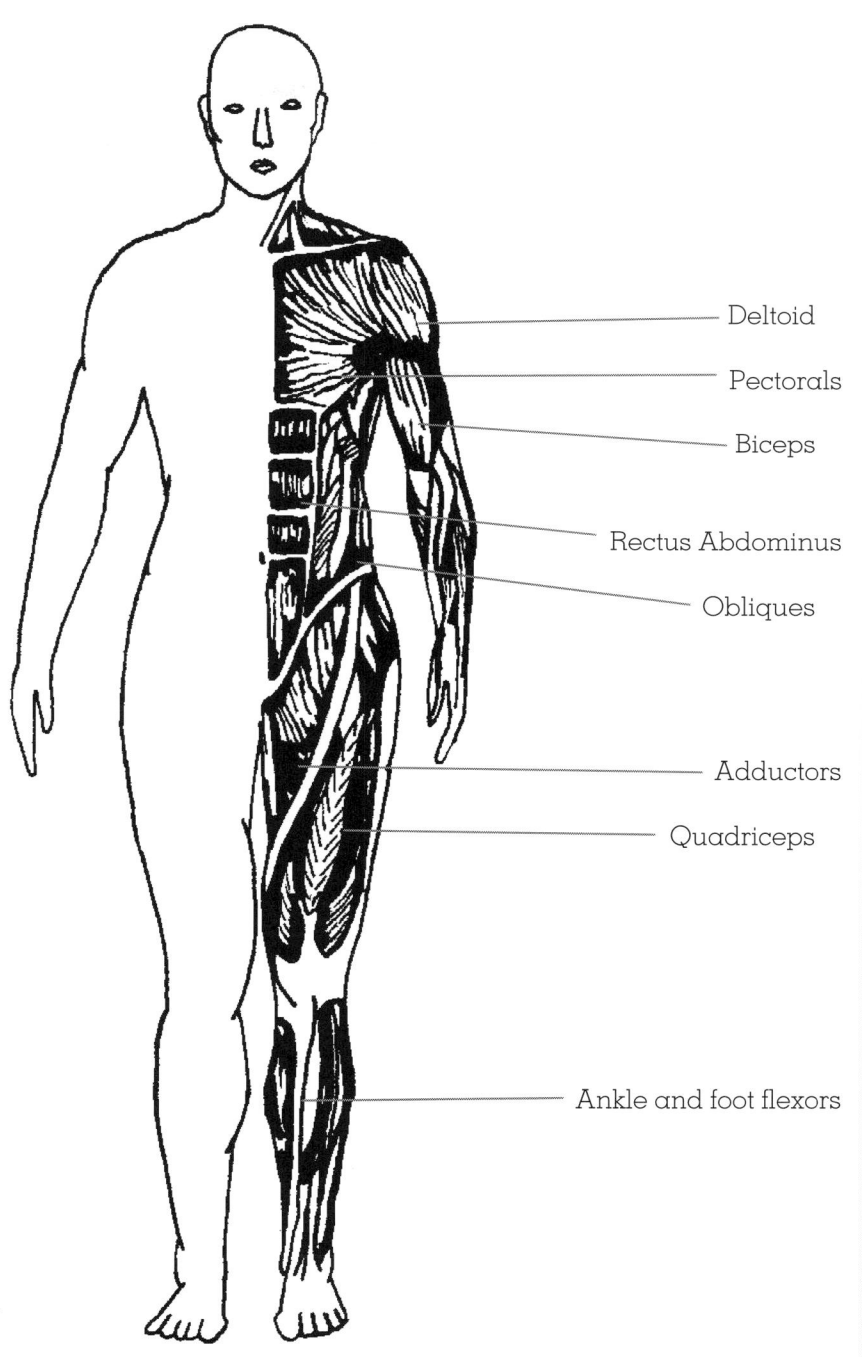

1. Quads: Leg press
2. Quads, hamstrings: Seated (or lying) leg curls
3. Quads, with an emphasis on strengthening knee area: Leg extensions
4. Quads: Squats
5. Chest: Push-ups
6. Chest: Machine chest press
7. Back: Pull-ups (with pull-up assist machine)
8. Back: Seated machine rows
9. Shoulders: Machine shoulder press or overhead seated dumbbell press
10. Biceps: Barbell curls with body bar
11. Triceps: Seated overhead tricep extensions
12. Abs: Crunches (four variations)

Reps and sets. How many sets and repetitions of each exercise should you do? In the beginning of your exercise program, you should try to do one set of 15 to 20 reps of each exercise. When you can do that "comfortably," work up to two sets of 15 to 20 reps. Between sets, always take a 30-second to one-minute rest to give your muscles a chance to recuperate. Where weights are used, start with light (three- to five-pound) weights. As you become used to the weight, add weight in three- to five-pound increments. However, do not increase weights more than once every three weeks. Remember, *increasing weight is not the goal*. It is far more important to isolate the function of the muscle so that it becomes toned and efficient.

When two sets of 15 to 20 reps is no longer challenging to you, you can mix up your workout a little more: Do one "warm-up" set of 15 to 20 reps of each exercise using a light weight, then do two to three "working" sets of 10 to 12 reps of each exercise with heavier weights (five to ten pounds heavier). As you increase the weight, you should decrease the reps. Furthermore, you should not bother doing more than three sets of any one exercise—it's a waste of time and effort. This is one of the instances when more is not necessarily better. It's just *more*.

Another way to add challenges to the basic workout is to add the following, more advanced exercises to the original workout:

1. Quads: Squats with body bar
2. Chest: Dumbbell chest press
3. Back: Lat pull-down and single-arm dumbbell rows on bench
4. Shoulders: Standing dumbbell lateral raises

5. Biceps: Standing alternating dumbbell curls
6. Triceps: Tricep kickbacks
7. Abs: Ab supersets

Ab Supersets. The most common abdominal exercises are crunches. People often confuse crunches with their popular predecessor, sit-ups. What's the difference between a sit-up and a crunch? In a crunch, after you lift your shoulder blades off the ground, you do not put them all the way back down again until you've completed all your reps.

Although the range of motion in a crunch is much smaller than in a sit-up, crunches are way more difficult. You may be able to do hundreds of sit-ups, but only a few crunches! As fitness professionals like to say about any exercise, if you do 'em wrong, you can do 'em all day long.

The idea behind crunches is to maintain continuous tension in the abdominal muscle. Doing so makes crunches much more effective than sit-ups—and that's what it's all about.

Furthermore, by limiting the range of motion, crunches are easier on your back than sit-ups. Think of a credit card that you bend slightly in one direction. What if you started bending it in the opposite direction—forward and back, forward and back? It would snap! Well, you don't want to do that to your back, do you?

In the descriptions below, we'll take you through four variations of the crunch, each one more difficult than the last. When you can complete two sets of 20 to 30 reps of each crunch easily, taking a rest of less than 30 seconds between sets (don't worry—it may take a while!), do one ab "superset": 20 to 30 reps of each type of crunch with *no* rest between variations. When you need to challenge yourself even more, try to do two to three supersets.

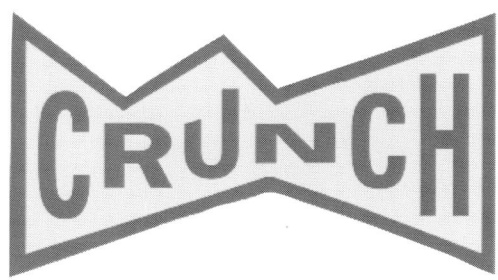

BEGINNER'S LUCK

HOW TO DO THE STRENGTH TRAINING EXERCISES

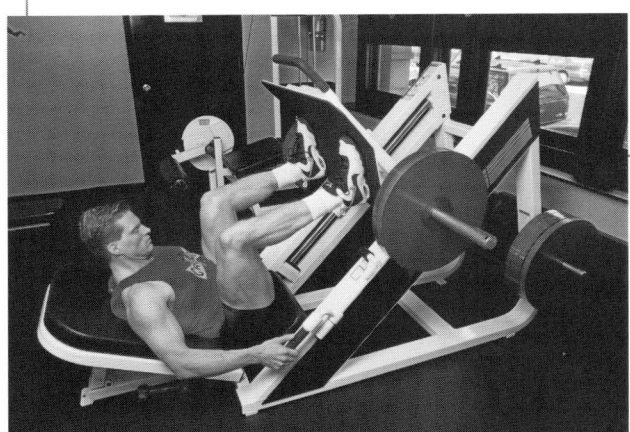

LEG PRESS

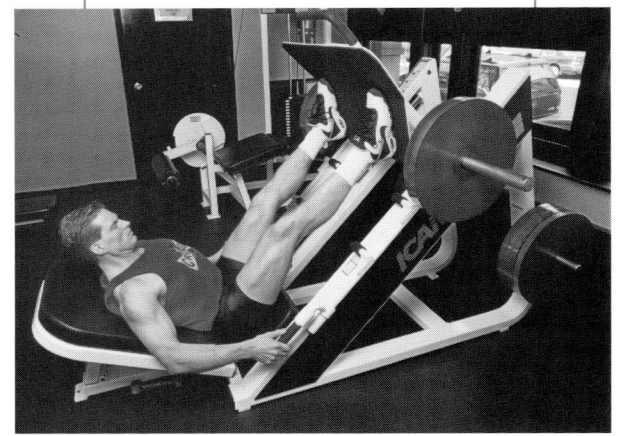

Sitting on the leg press, grab the handles at your sides. To start, your knees and upper legs should be at a 90 degree angle to your torso. You may position your feet low on the platform or high, shoulder-width apart. Press the weight up until your legs are fully extended, but don't lock your knees (as in the "bad form" photo).

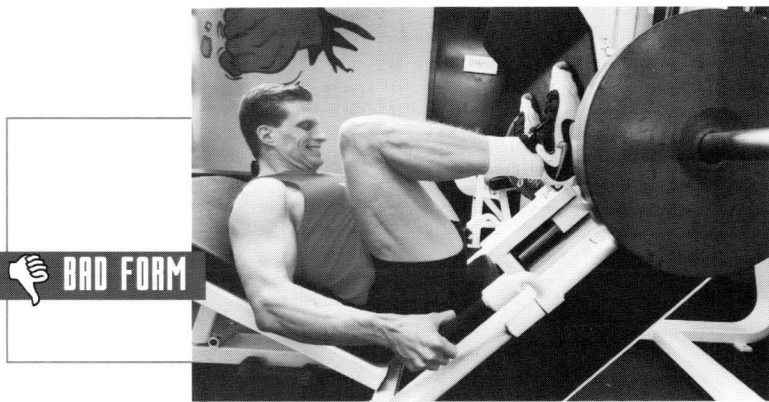

BAD FORM

THE WORKOUT

QUAD STRETCH

Between sets of leg exercises, stretch your quads. Grab a piece of equipment (or other stationary object) with one hand, and grab your opposite ankle with the other hand. Pull up slightly, keeping your thighs even with each other. (In the bad form photo, notice how the thigh is raised up and out.) Hold for 15 seconds and switch sides.

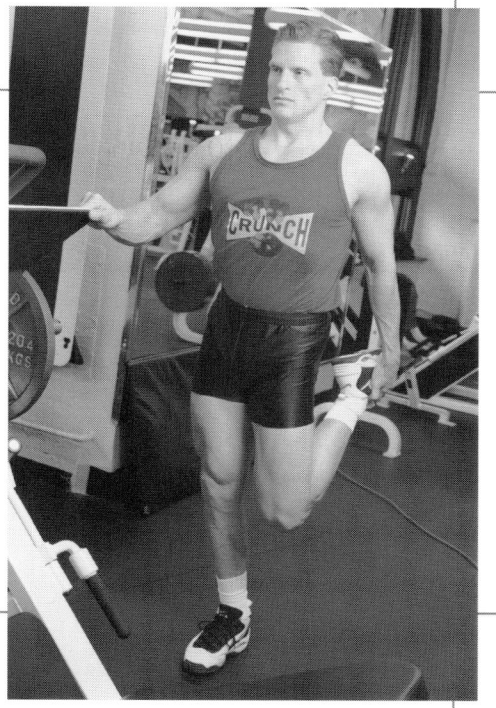

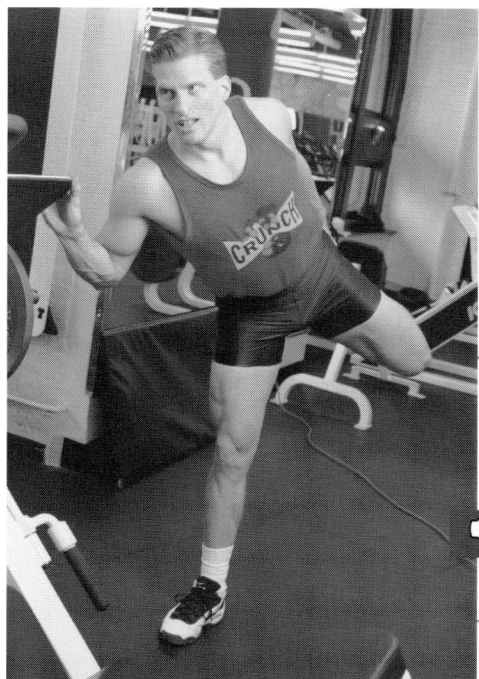

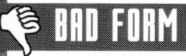
BAD FORM

BEGINNER'S LUCK

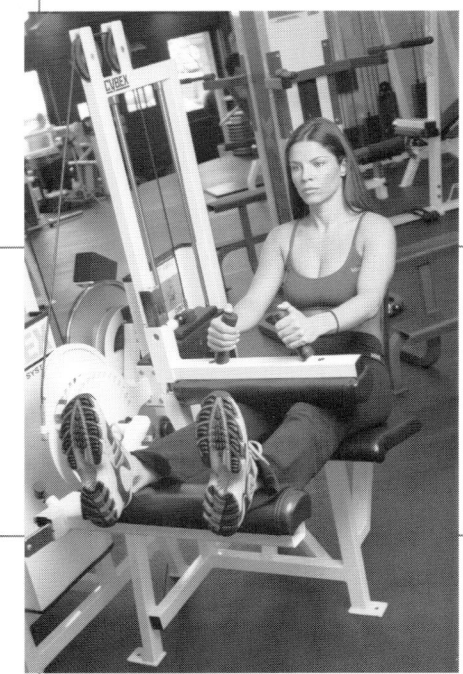
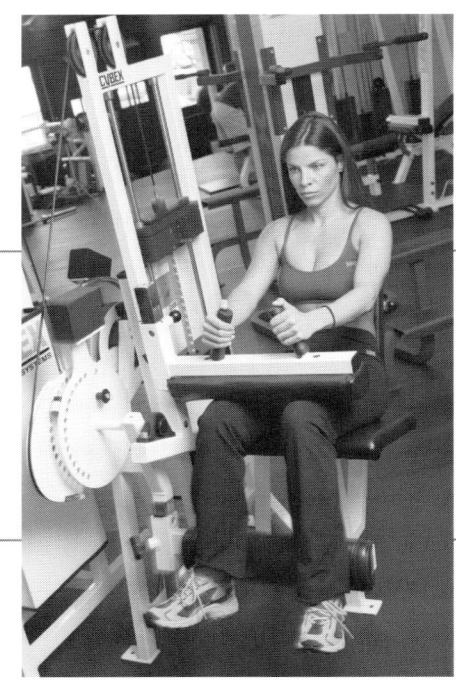

SEATED LEG CURLS

Sit on the leg curl machine and hold the bars at your sides. The pad should rest on the back of your ankles. Align the axis pin to the rear of your knee by adjusting your seat back accordingly. *This is very important!* If the axis pin is not aligned correctly, you could hurt your knees. Point your toes toward the ceiling and keep your back slightly flexed so that your lower back is *not* touching the seat back. Press the pad down so that a 90 degree angle is formed between your upper and lower legs.

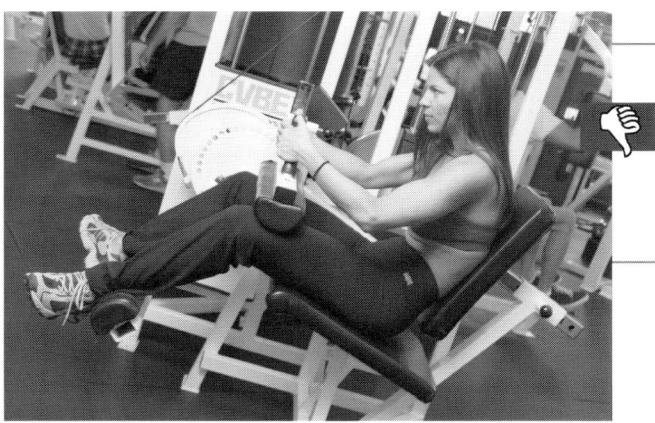

BAD FORM

THE WORKOUT

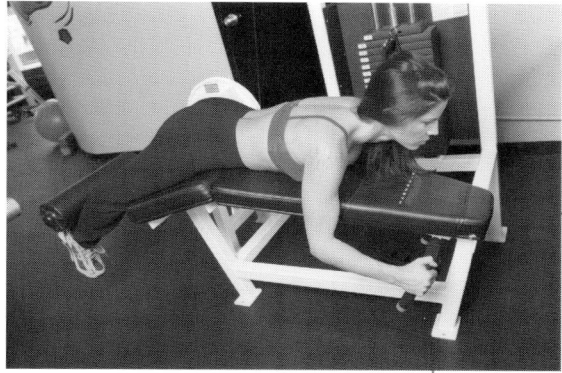

LYING LEG CURL

If your gym doesn't have a seated leg curl, it probably has a lying leg curl. Either machine is fine. If you're using a lying leg curl, lie on the bench with your face down and with the pad resting behind your ankles. Grab the handles. Keep your legs aligned with your feet and hips, and keep your abs tight. Don't bring the pad all the way down between reps.

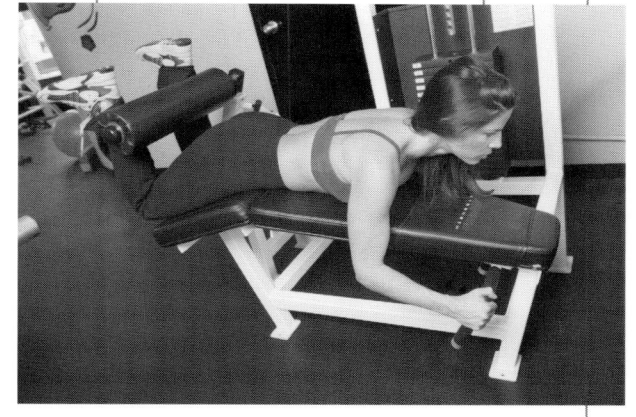

In the bad form photo, notice how the back is swayed and the head is up.

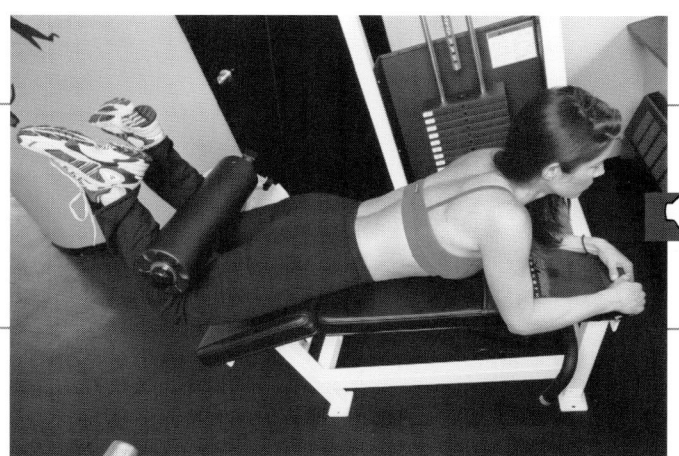

BAD FORM

BEGINNER'S LUCK

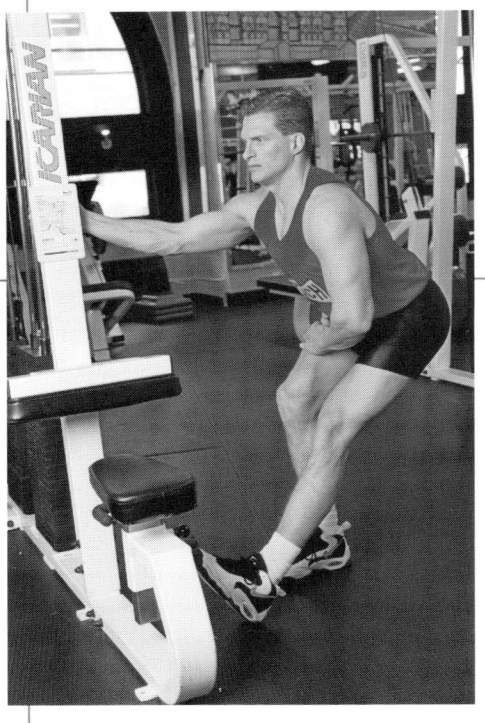

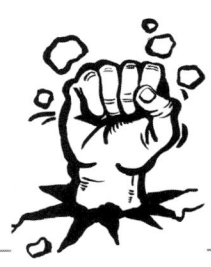

HAMSTRING STRETCH

Between sets of hamstring exercises, stretch your hams. Grab onto a stable object. Bend one leg and position the other leg out in front of you. Lean back. Keep the free hand on the opposite thigh. Keep your chest up and keep your torso upright. Repeat on opposite side.

In the bad form photo, notice how the shoulders are curled in. Avoid this position!

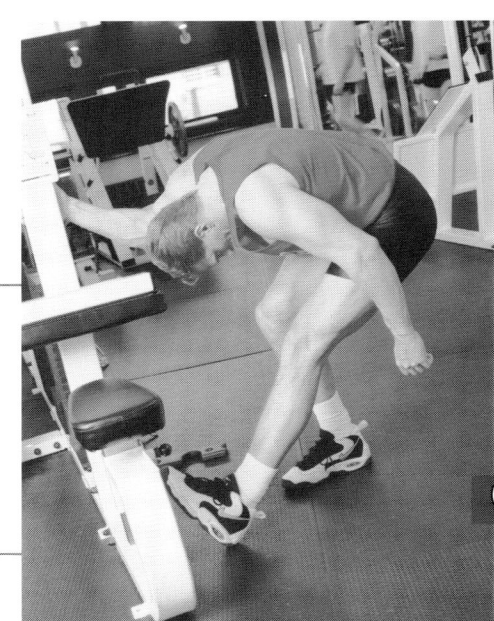

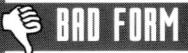

THE WORKOUT

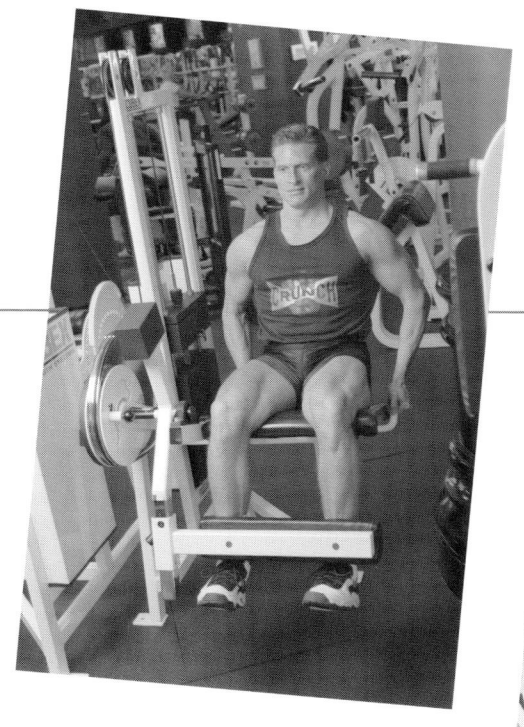

LEG EXTENSIONS

Sit on the leg extension machine and grab the bars with both hands. Make sure the axis pin on the machine is aligned with the rear of your knee joint by adjusting the seat back accordingly. This is very important to avoid injury to your knee! The shin pad should rest just above the front ankles. Extend your legs fully, but do not lock your knee at the top. Do not bring the weight all the way down between reps.

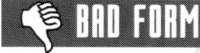
BAD FORM

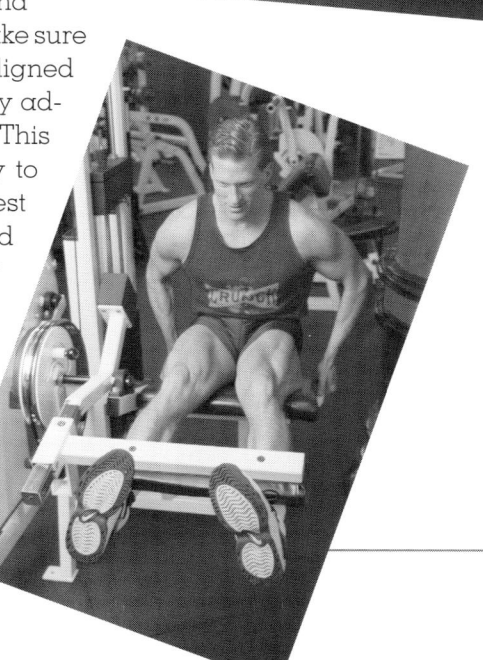

BEGINNER'S LUCK

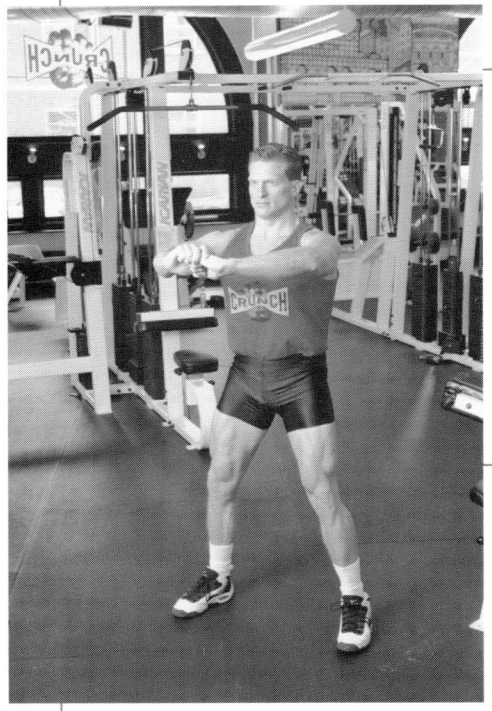

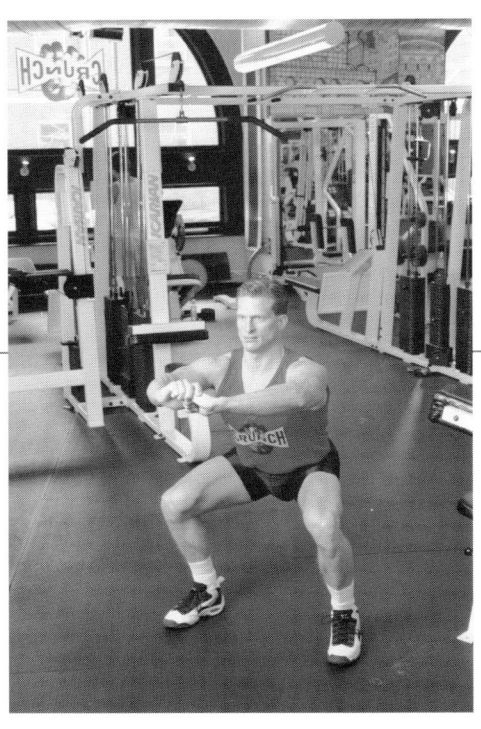

SQUATS

Stand with your feet shoulder-width apart and your feet slightly turned out. Put your hands out in front of you, and turn your palms outward. As you squat down, do not extend your knees over your toes. Keep your back straight and your head up. Think of sitting back into a chair—squat down directly; don't go forward. You want your thighs to become almost parallel to the floor.

BAD FORM

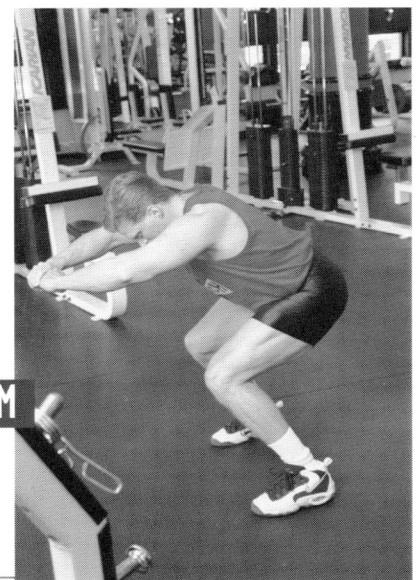

THE WORKOUT

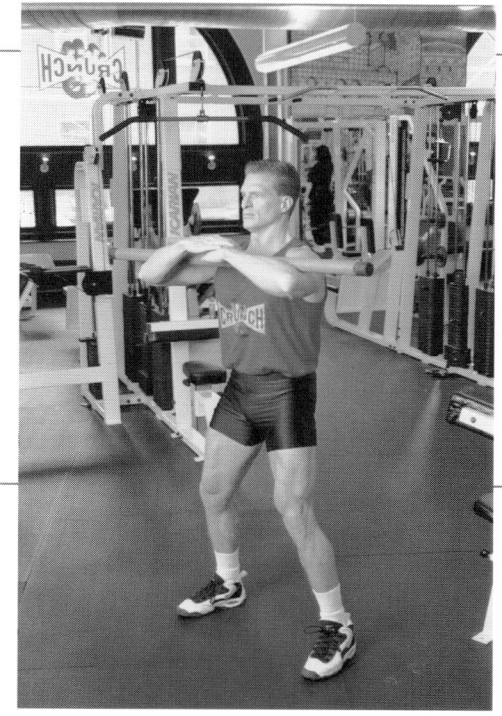

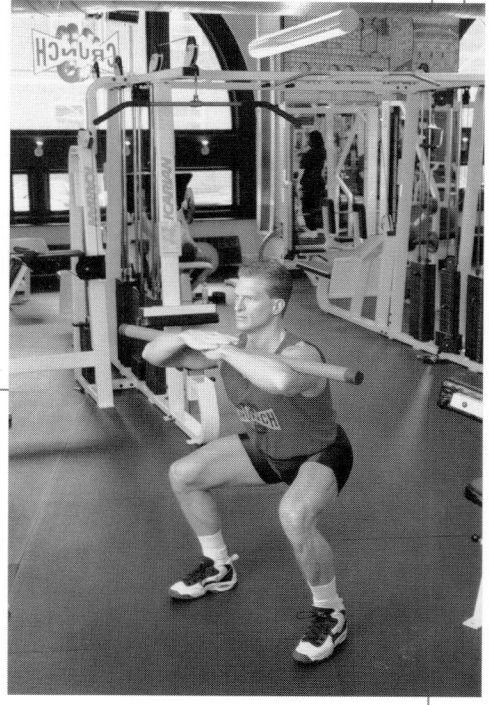

SQUATS WITH BODY BAR

Perform squats as described above, only cradle a body bar in your arms.
Do not hold the body bar in back of your head—doing so pulls you down and is very bad for your spine and neck.

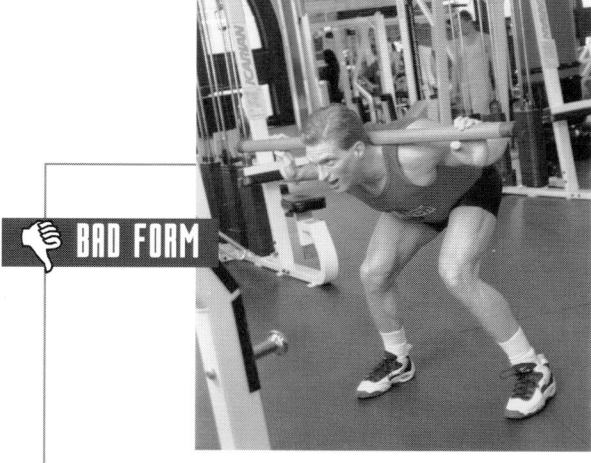

BAD FORM

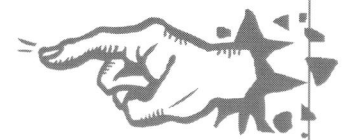

55

BEGINNER'S LUCK

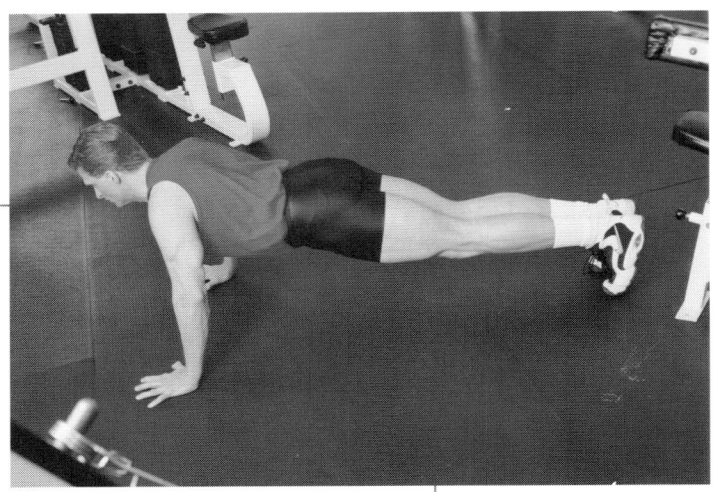

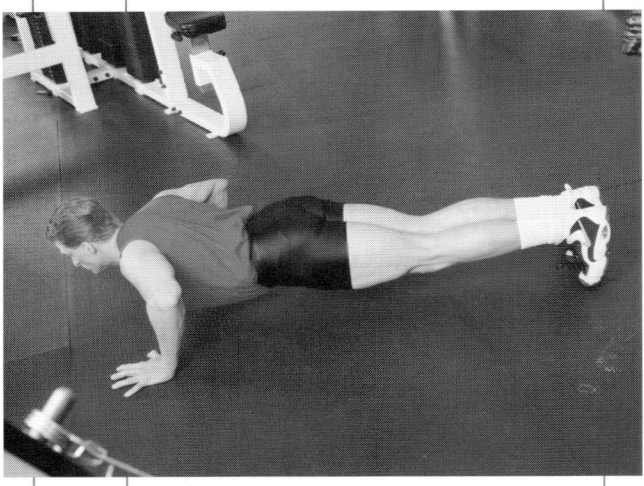

PUSH-UPS

You can do these from your knees, with your feet in the air, or from your toes. In either case, place your hands slightly wider than shoulder-width apart. Make sure you look forward, not down, as you do the push-ups. Keep your abs tight, your back flat (not swayed), and your head up. While push-ups mainly work the chest muscles, they also work the triceps and abs.

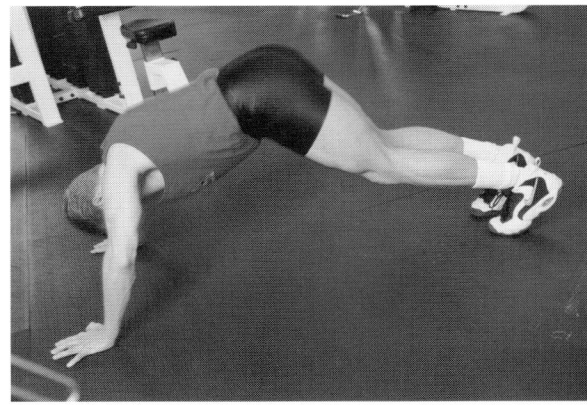

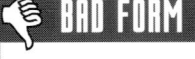

THE WORKOUT

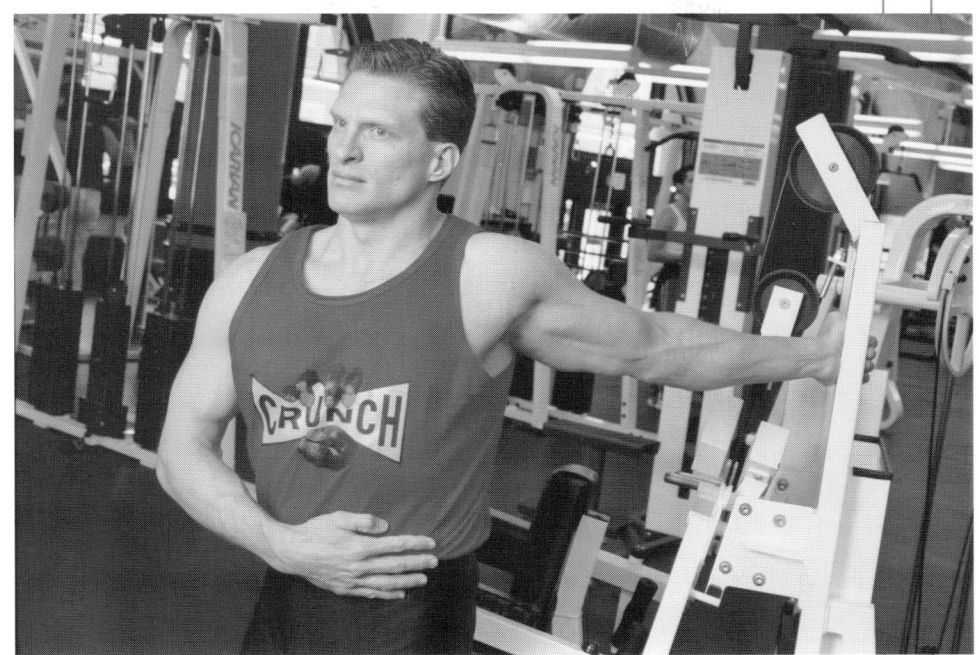

PEC STRETCH

Between sets of pectoral exercises, stretch your pecs. Grab a secure object with one hand. With your arm outstretched, slightly turn away from the arm (do not turn excessively). Do not turn your shoulder in. Hold the stretch for 15 seconds and repeat on other side.

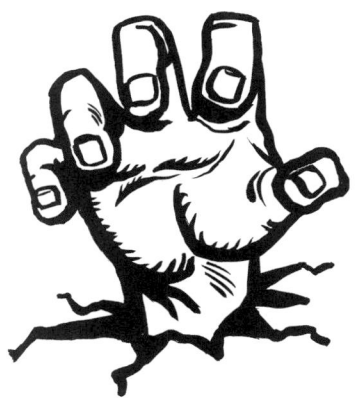

BEGINNER'S LUCK

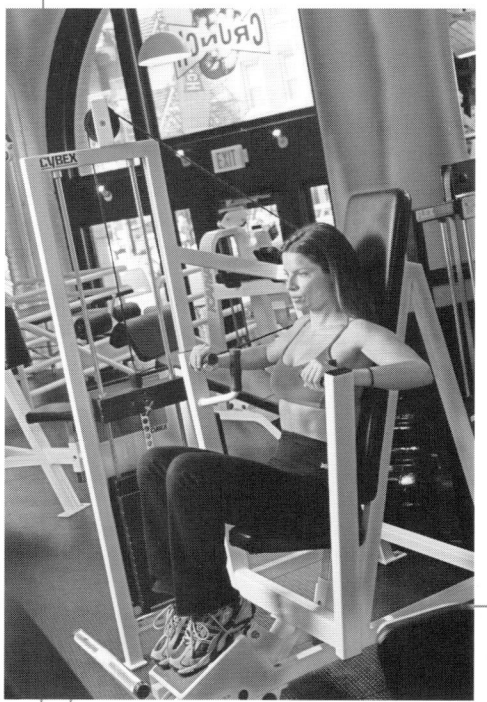 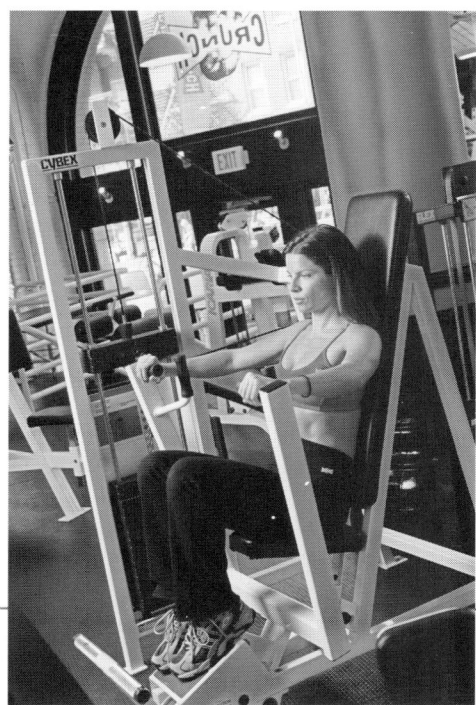

MACHINE CHEST PRESS

Keeping your shoulder blades back against the pad at all times, press the weight out. Do not lock your elbows at the top and do not bring your elbows back beyond a 90 degree angle with your torso (as shown in the bad form shot).

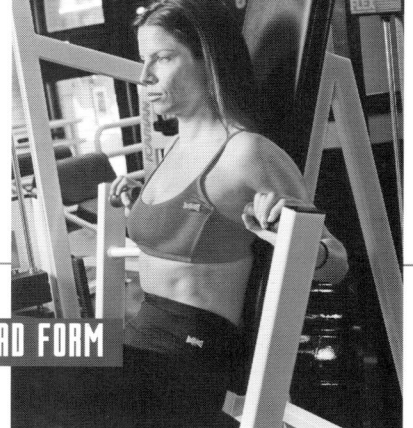 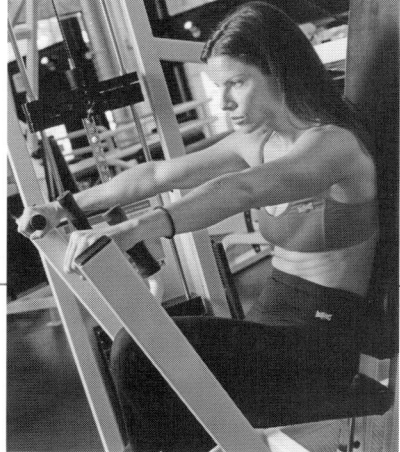

BAD FORM

THE WORKOUT

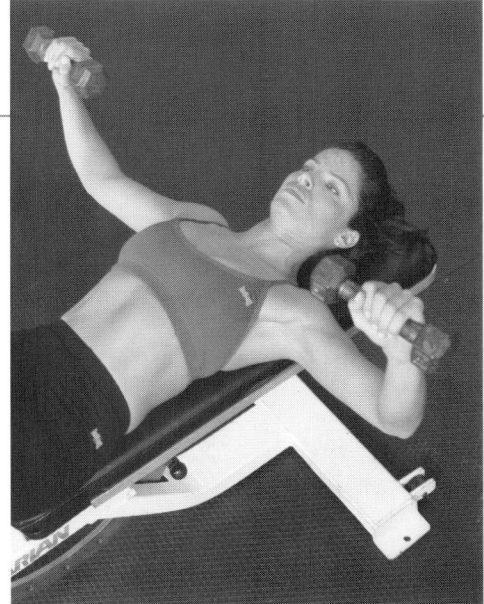

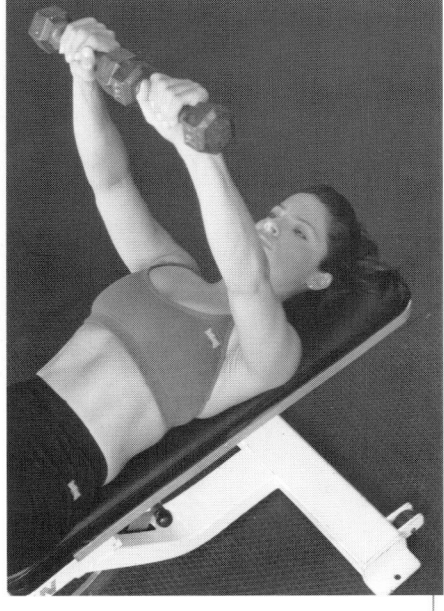

DUMBBELL CHEST PRESS

Lie on your back on the bench. Grasp dumbbells in each hand with palms facing away from you. To start, hold the dumbbells in fully extended arms over the mid-line of your chest. Bring the dumbbells down, bending your elbows. Do not drop your elbows below your body at the bottom, and do not lock your elbows at the top.

👎 **BAD FORM**

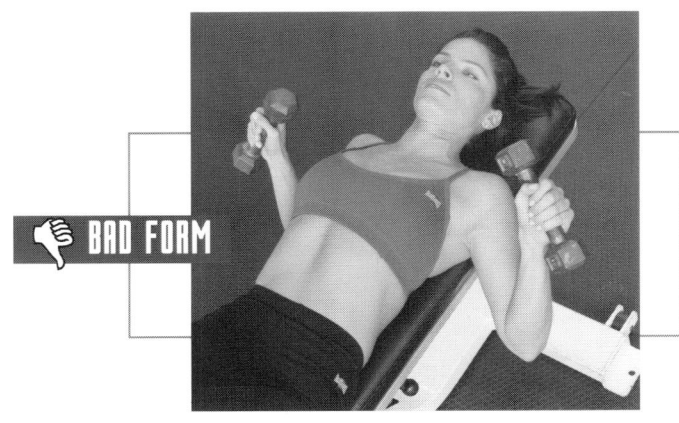

BEGINNER'S LUCK

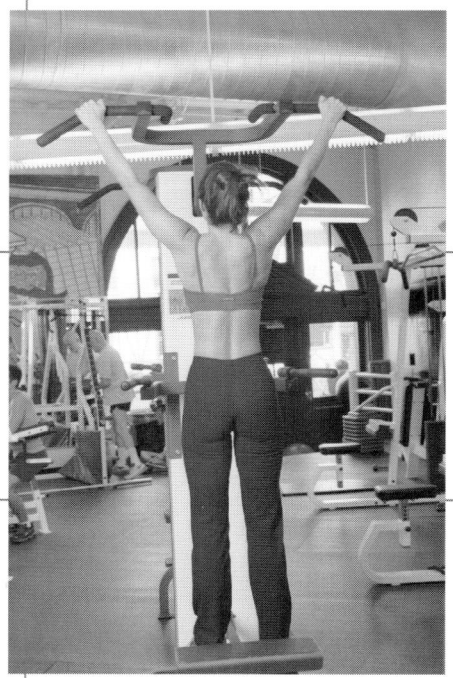
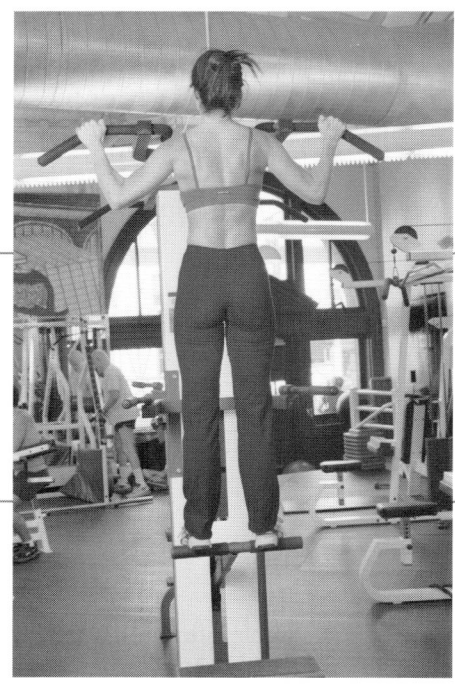

PULL-UPS (WITH PULL-UP ASSIST MACHINE)

The weight in this machine is designed to counterbalance your body weight. Start off with a heavy weight and gradually decrease the weight until you're able to do pull-ups with no weight at all.

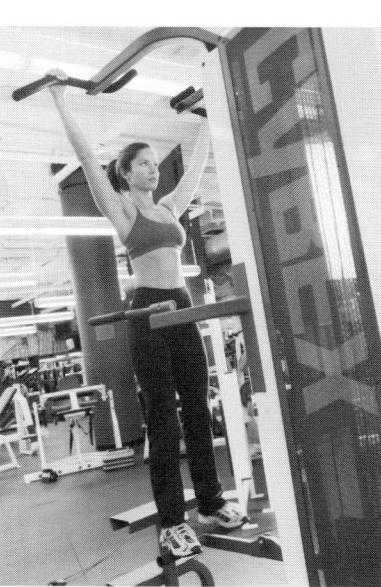

Grasp the pull-up bar in a wide grip with palms facing outward. Lead with your chest as you pull yourself up. Keep your head up.

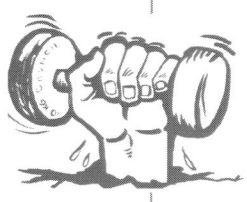

THE WORKOUT

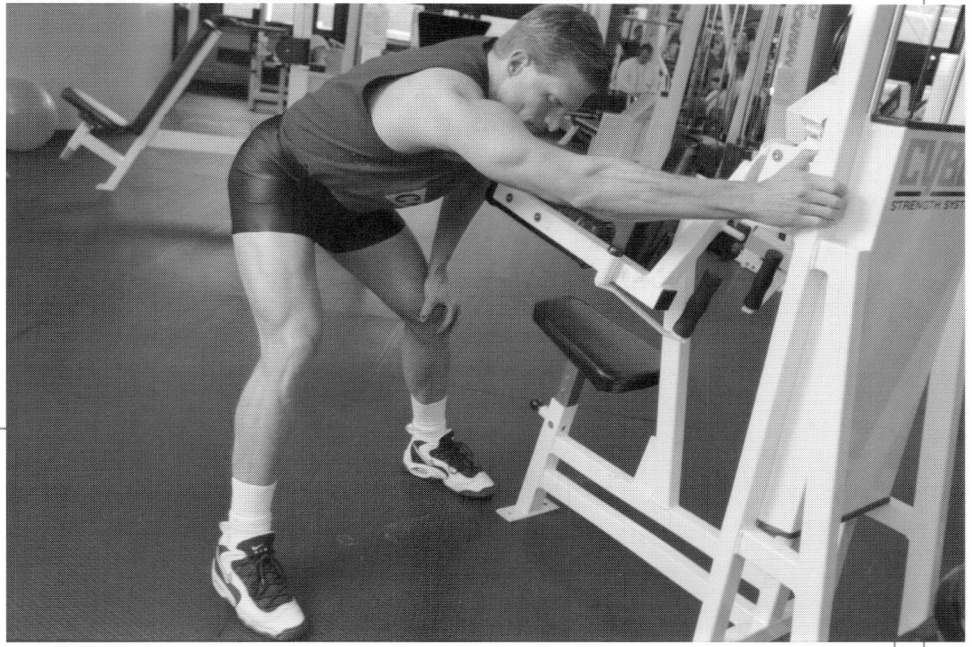

LAT STRETCH

Between sets of back exercises, stretch your back muscles. With your knees slightly bent and your back flat, grab a stationary object with one arm and lean back. Feel the stretch in your back. Hold for 15 seconds and repeat on other side.

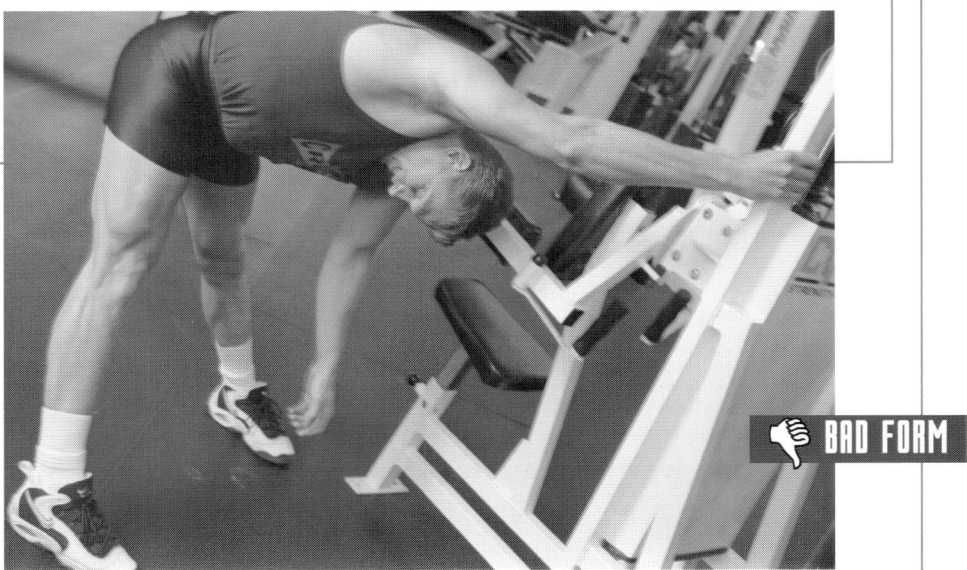

BAD FORM

BEGINNER'S LUCK

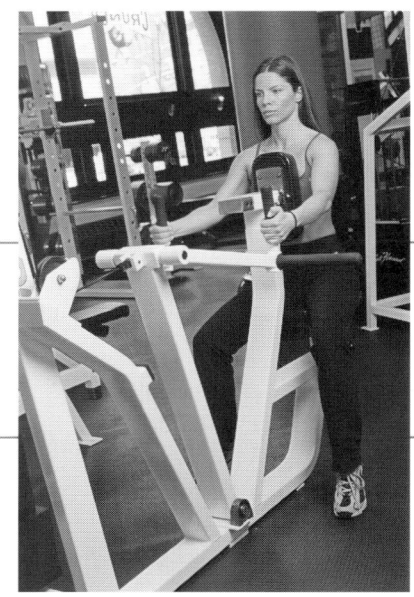 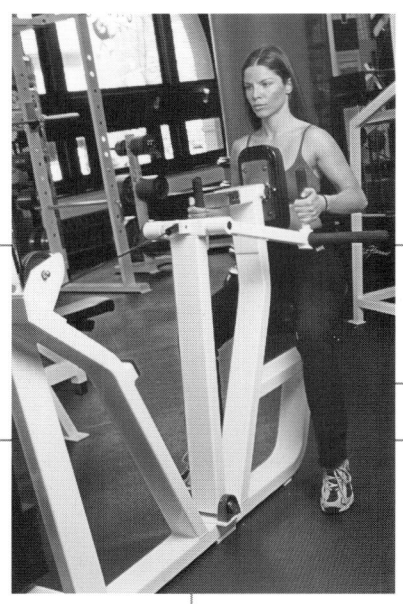

SEATED MACHINE ROW

Keep your back straight and support yourself, rather than resting your chest on the chest pad. Don't round your shoulders forward. Grabbing the handles low, drive your elbows back, rather than pulling back with your hands.

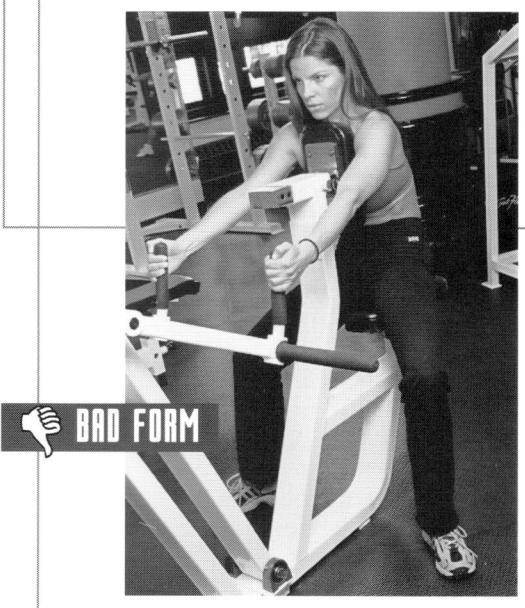 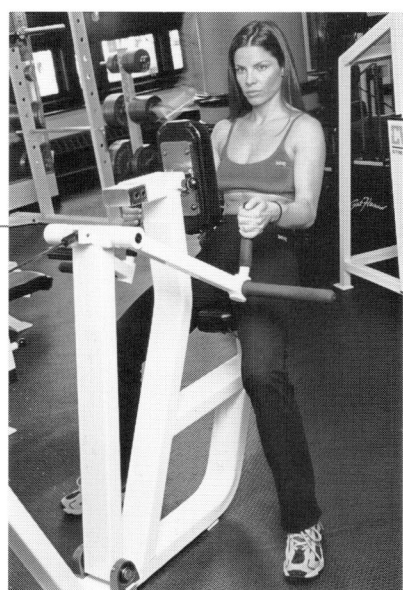

BAD FORM

THE WORKOUT

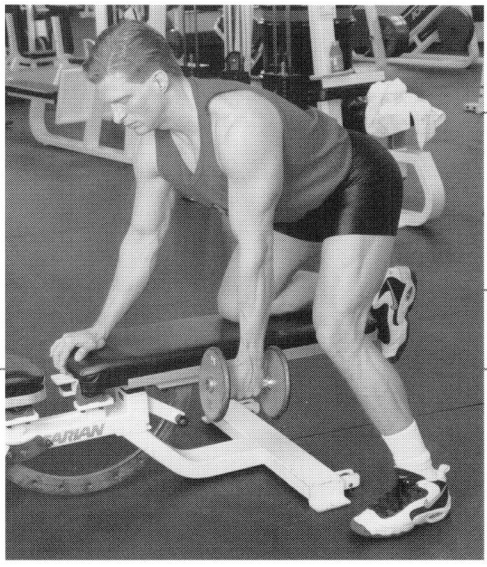

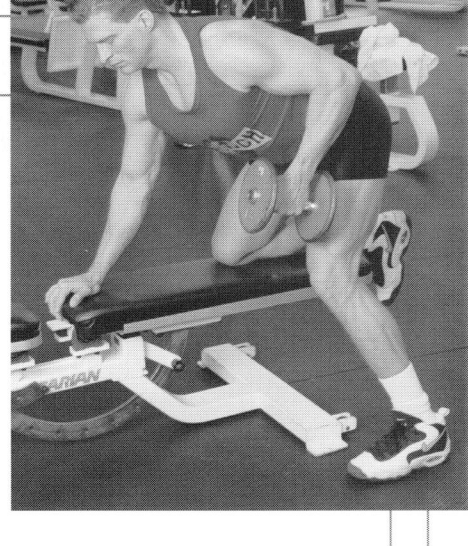

SINGLE-ARM DUMBBELL ROWS ON BENCH

Hold a dumbbell in one arm and place the opposite arm and knee on the bench. Your weight should be evenly distributed among your kneeling leg, your standing leg, and your arm on the bench. Bring the dumbbell up toward your hip (do not bring it up all the way to your rib cage). Keep your back flat.

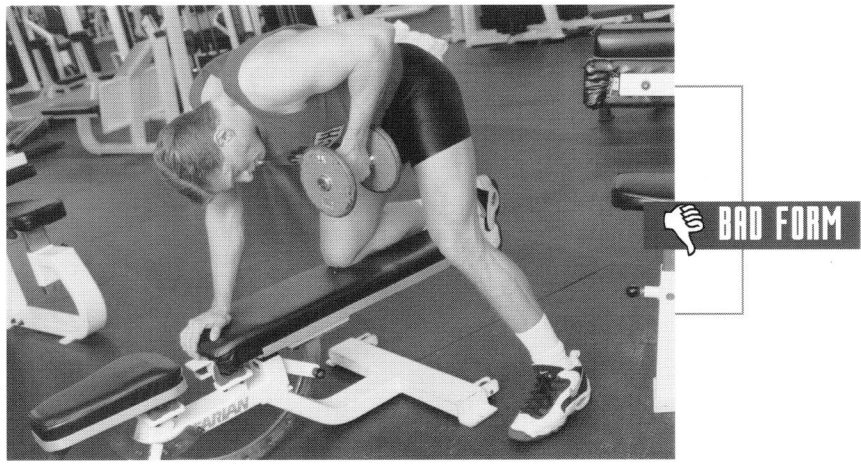

BAD FORM

BEGINNER'S LUCK

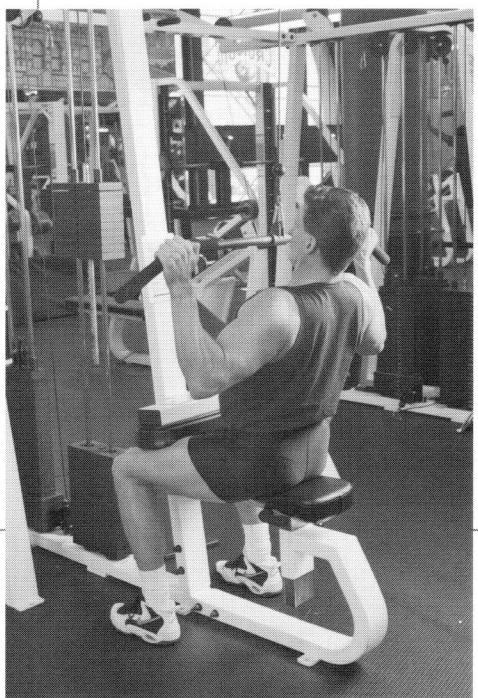

LAT PULL-DOWNS

Sit with the pad above your thighs. With a shoulder-width overgrip, pull the bar to the middle of your chest. Keep your back straight. Do *not* pull down or press down behind your head—you can injure your shoulder. Unfortunately, this is a very common mistake among gym members.

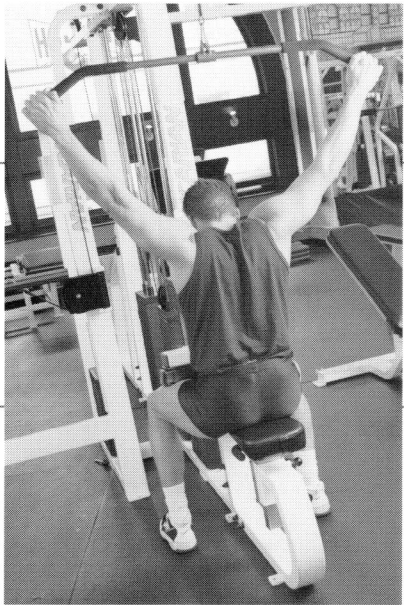

👎 BAD FORM

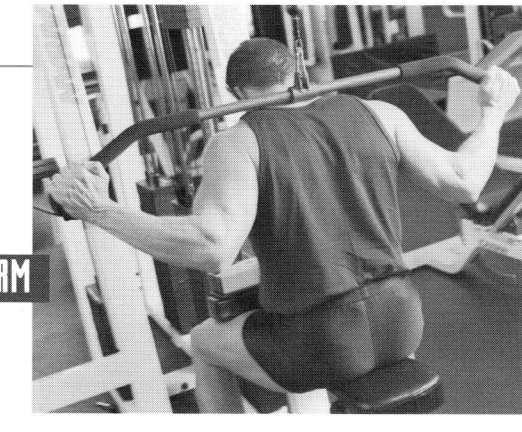

THE WORKOUT

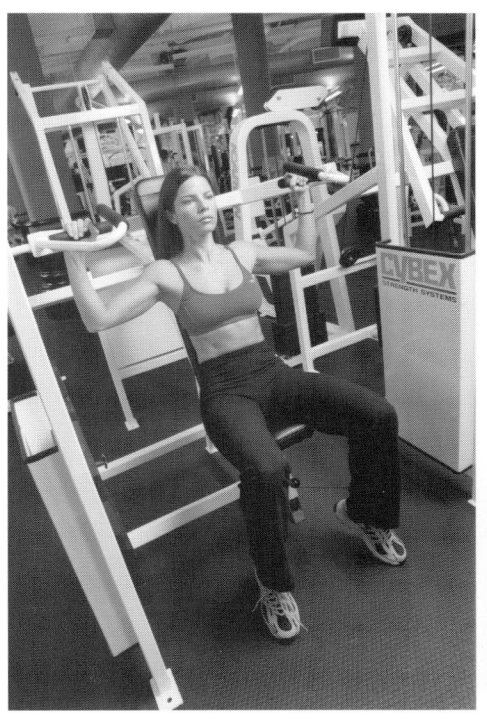
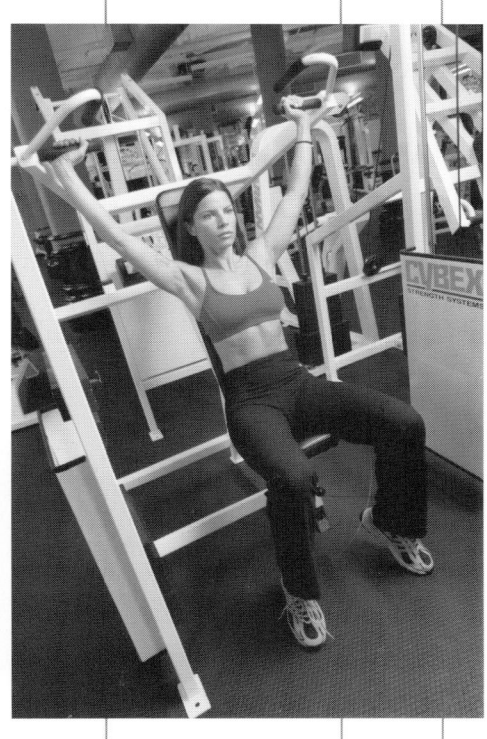

MACHINE SHOULDER PRESS

Seated, grasp the handles while keeping a slight forward bend in your elbows. Raise your arms without locking them at the top. Do not drop the weight all the way down between reps. (Notice how the elbows are locked in the bad form photo.)

BAD FORM

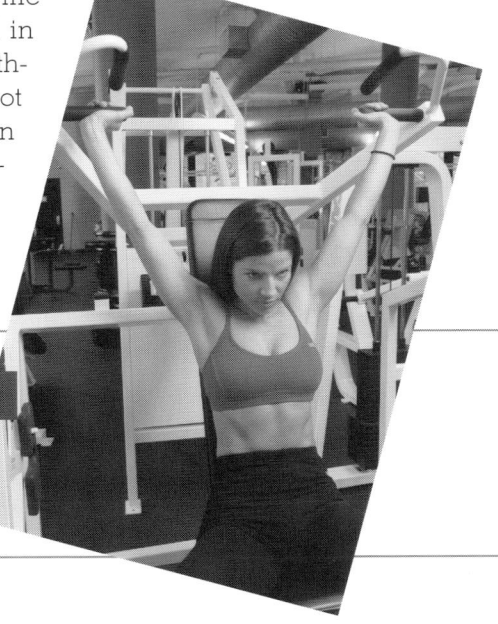

BEGINNER'S LUCK

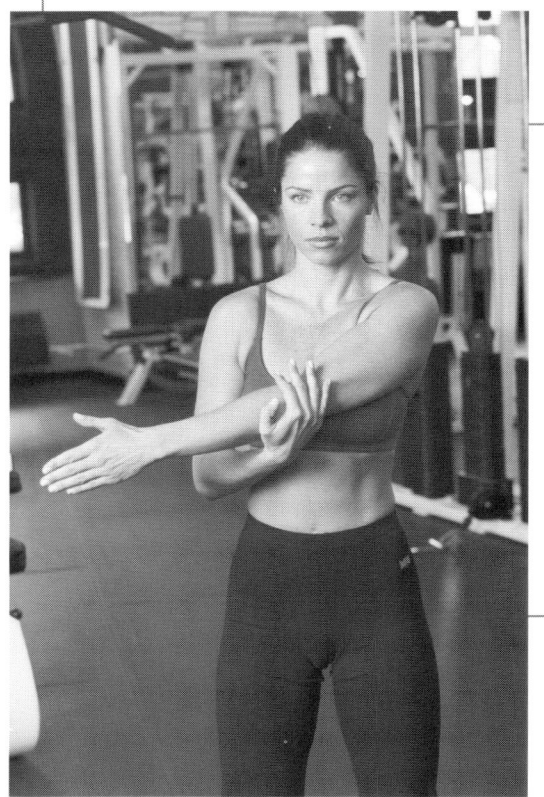

SHOULDER STRETCH

Between sets of shoulder exercises, stretch your shoulder muscles. Hold one bent elbow with your opposite hand and slightly pull it across your body. Keep your shoulder relaxed. Hold for 15 seconds and repeat on opposite side.

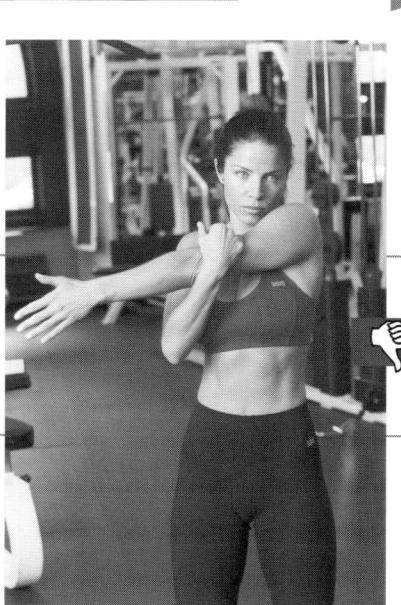

BAD FORM

THE WORKOUT

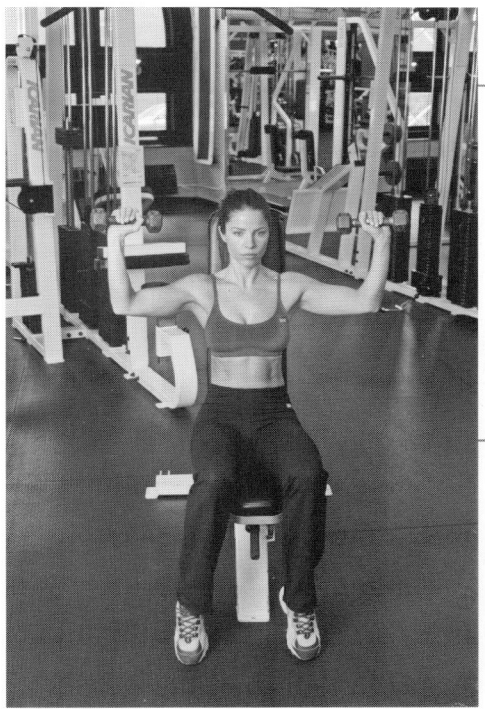

OVERHEAD SEATED DUMBBELL PRESS

Sit on the bench with your feet flat on the floor. Hold the dumbbells out to your sides at ear level. Raise the dumbbells overhead, being careful not to lock your elbows at the top. Keep the space between your ears and elbows as open as possible.

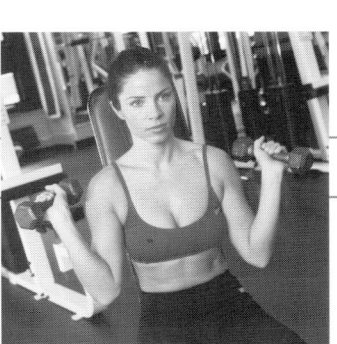

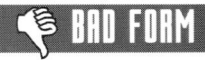
BAD FORM

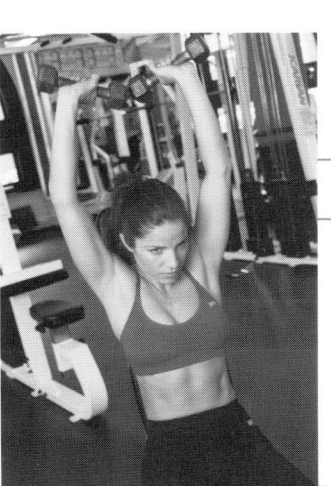

BEGINNER'S LUCK

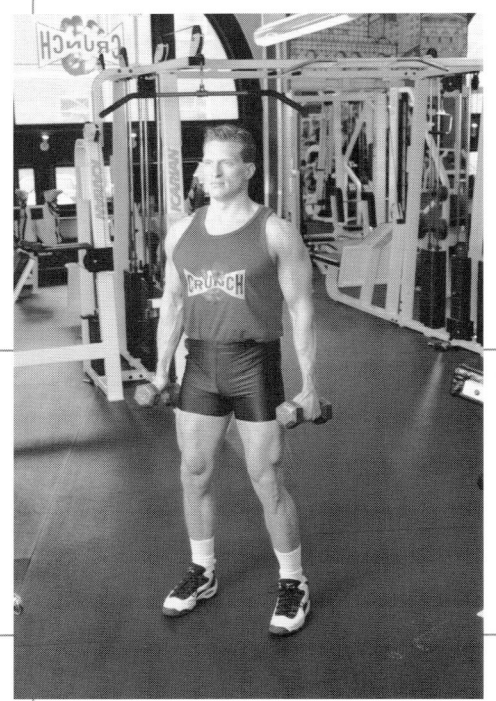
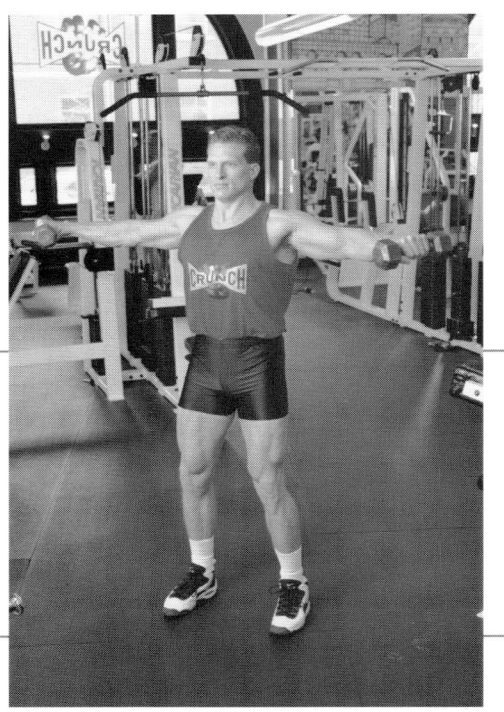

STANDING DUMBBELL LATERAL RAISES

Stand straight with your feet shoulder-width apart and knees slightly bent. Hold the dumbbells in your hands with your palms facing down, elbows slightly bent, and arms in front of your body. Raise your arms slowly up to the shoulder, exhaling as you do so. Hold for two counts and slowly return to starting position, inhaling slowly. Do not raise the dumbbells over your shoulders, which will place stress on the shoulders and may injure the rotator cuff. Concentrate on moving your arms out laterally before lifting them straight up.

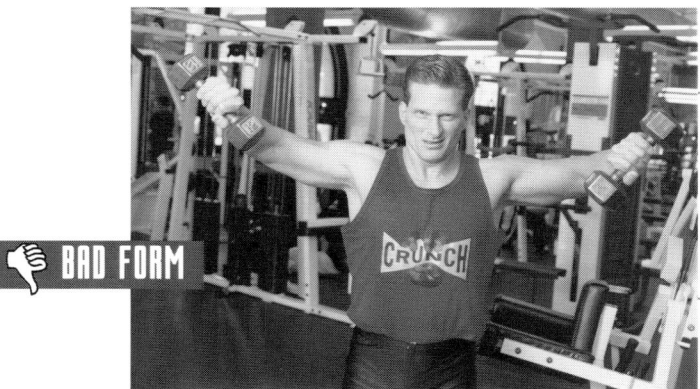

👎 BAD FORM

THE WORKOUT

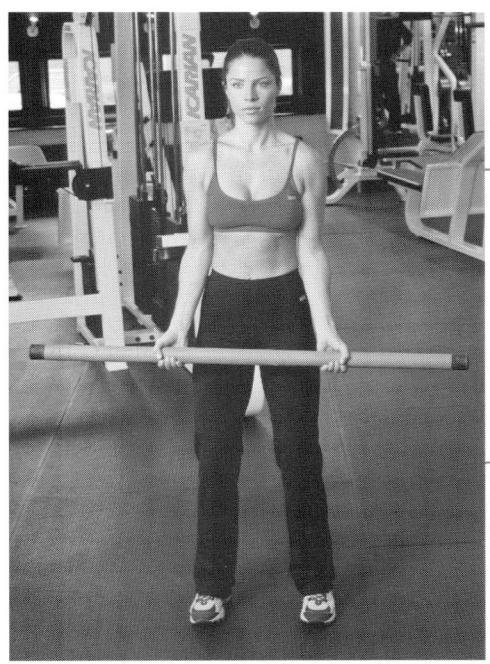 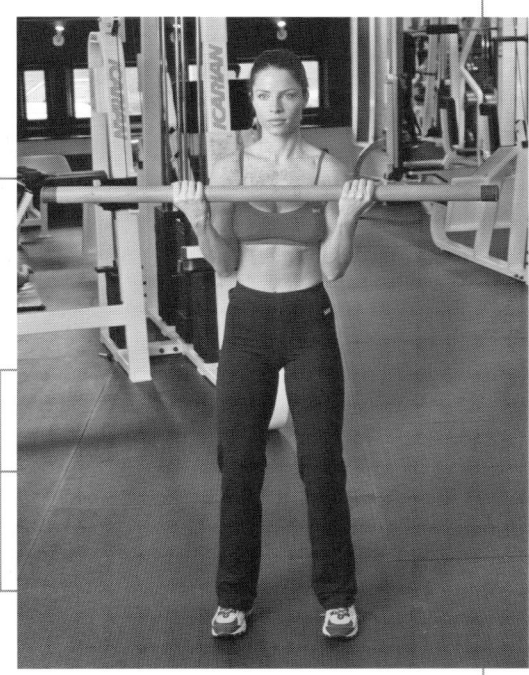

BARBELL CURL WITH BODY BAR

Stand straight with your feet shoulder-width apart. Hold the barbell in front of you with a slightly wider than shoulder-width underhand grip. Lift bar to shoulder level and slowly lower down again. Do not curl your wrist.

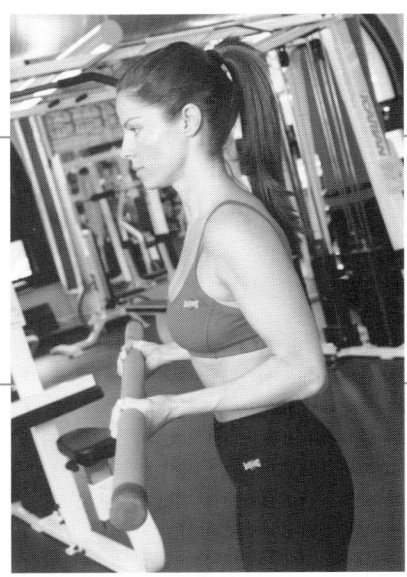 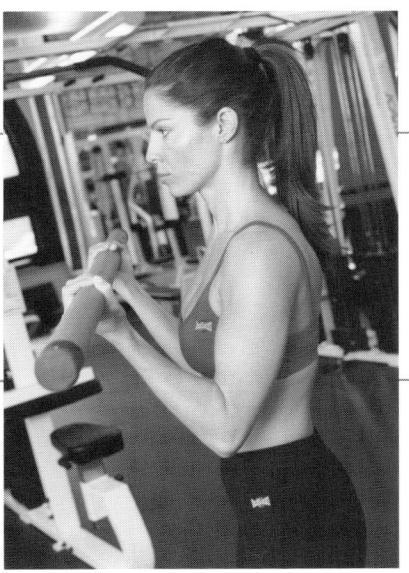

BEGINNER'S LUCK

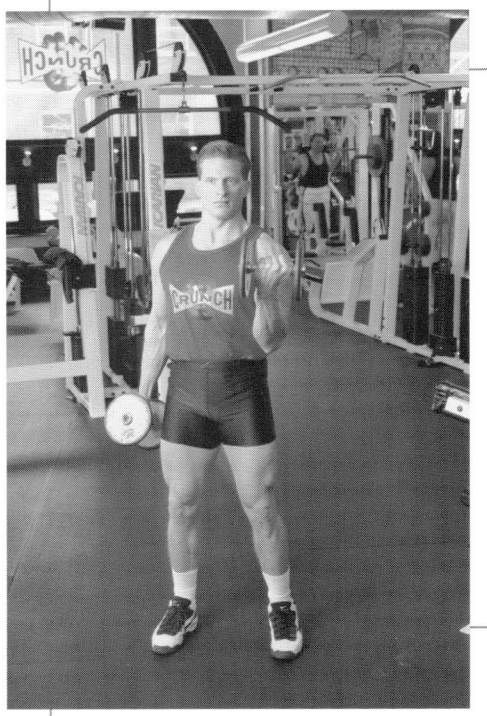

STANDING ALTERNATING DUMBBELL CURLS

Stand, holding dumbbells in each hand at your sides so that your palms face your legs. Raise one dumbbell at a time to your chest. As the dumbbell clears your leg, turn your wrist so that your palm faces your body, and turn your wrist back again on its way down. Perform this exercise in a slow and controlled motion. Do not switch arms until the one arm has completed the motion.

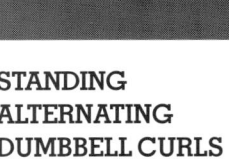
BAD FORM

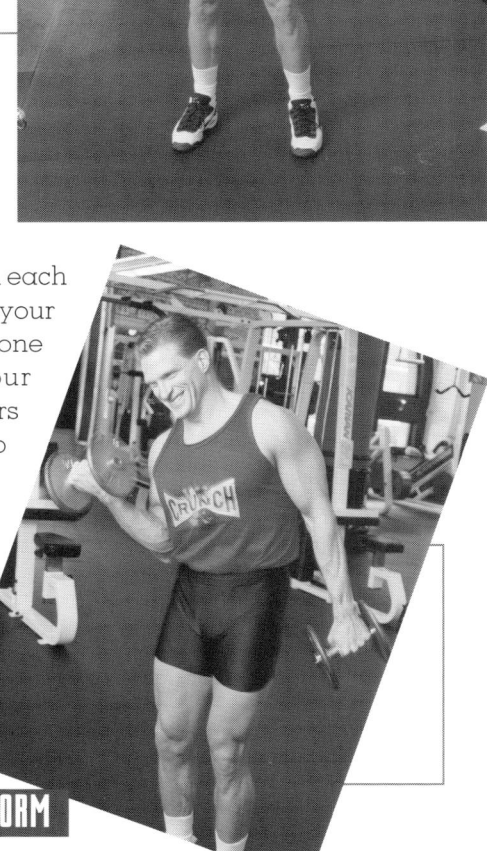

THE WORKOUT

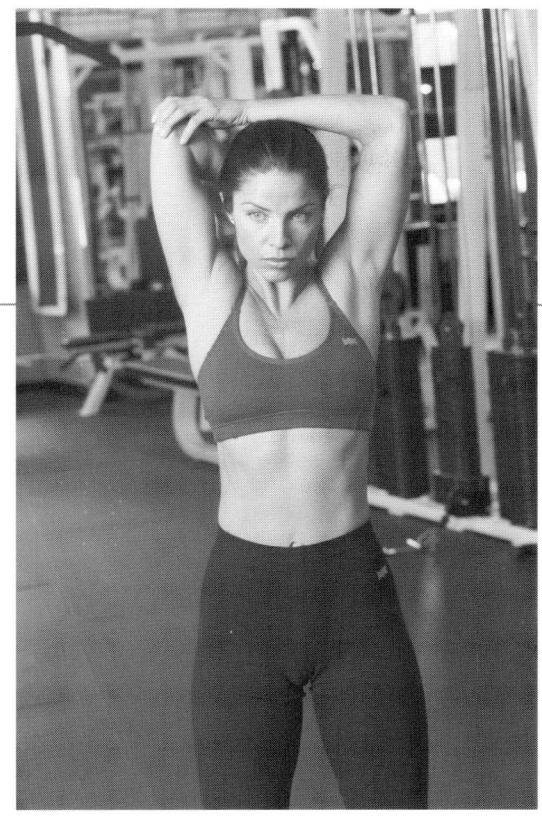

OVERHEAD TRICEP STRETCH

Between sets of tricep exercises, stretch your triceps. Grab one elbow behind your head with the opposite hand. Do not yank your body to the side. Hold and repeat on the opposite side.

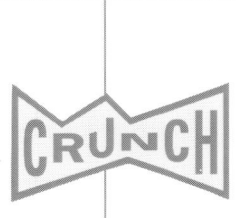

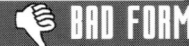 BAD FORM

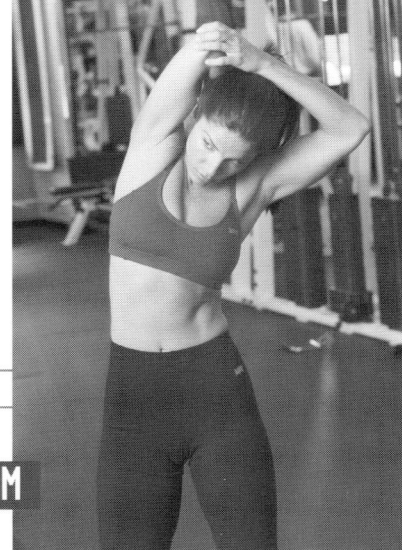

BEGINNER'S LUCK

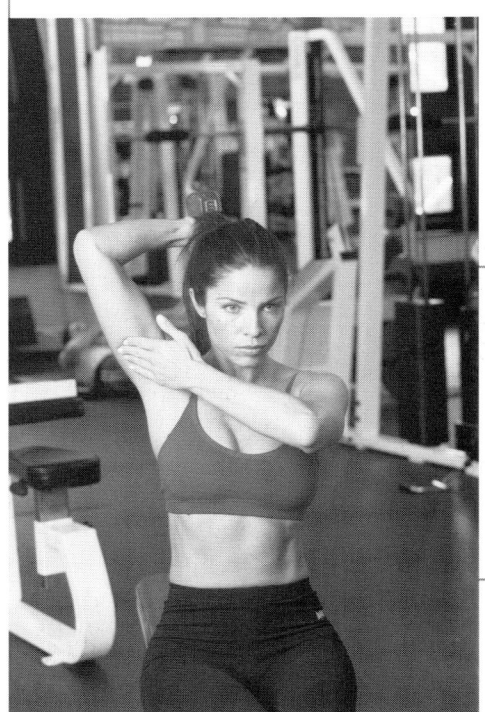
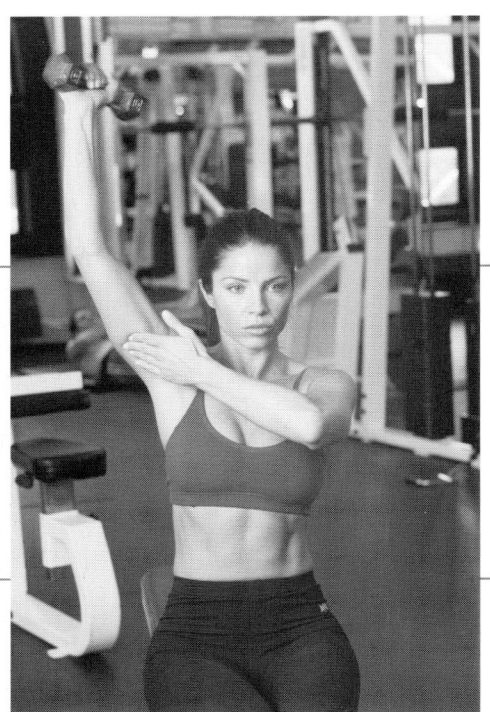

SEATED OVERHEAD TRICEP EXTENSION

Hold a dumbbell in one arm that is fully extended over your head. Bend your elbow back, bringing the dumbbell back behind your head. Keep your wrist straight. You can support the arm with your other hand. Repeat with the opposite arm.

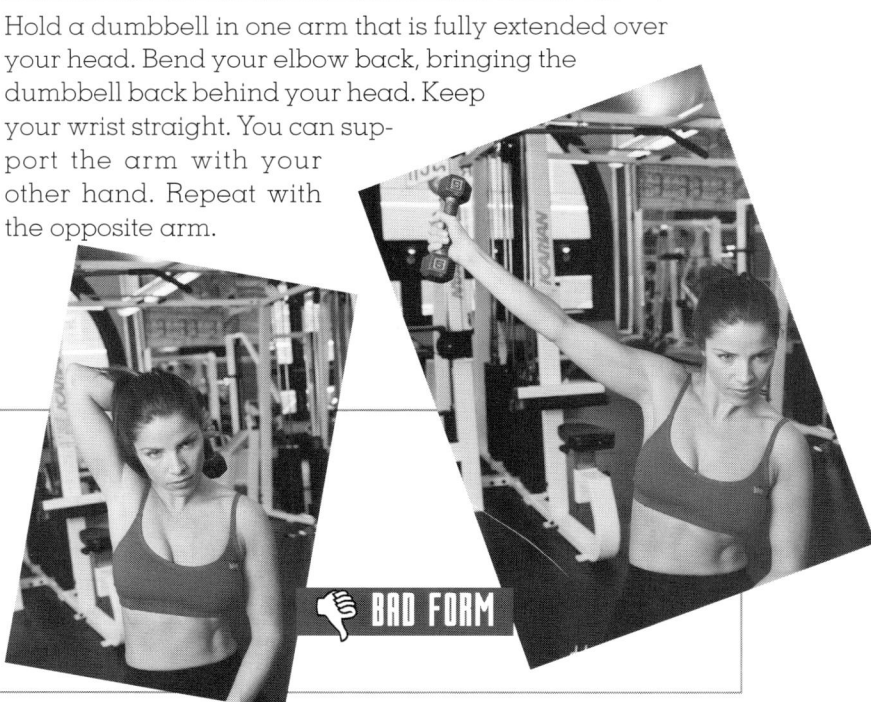

👎 BAD FORM

THE WORKOUT

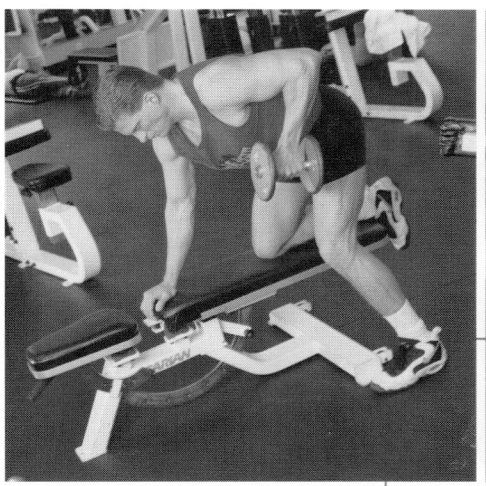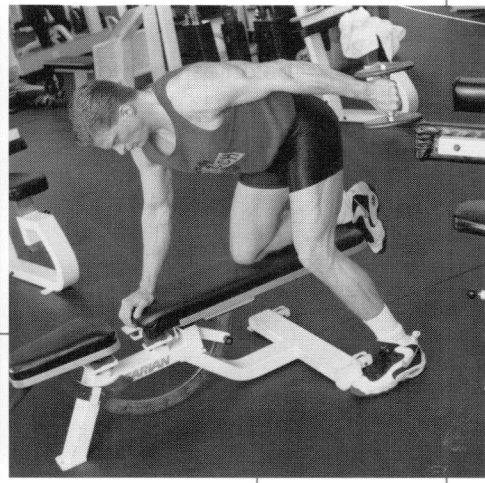

TRICEP KICKBACKS

Hold a dumbbell in one arm with your elbow bent and place the opposite arm and knee on the bench. Your weight should be evenly distributed among your kneeling leg, your standing leg, and your arm on the bench. Extend your forearm out behind you to a fully extended position, but *do not swing* your arm back. Repeat with the other arm.

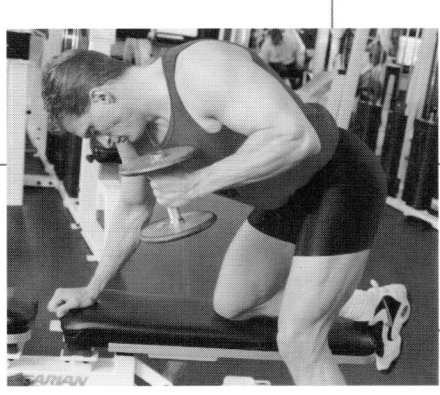

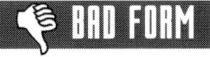

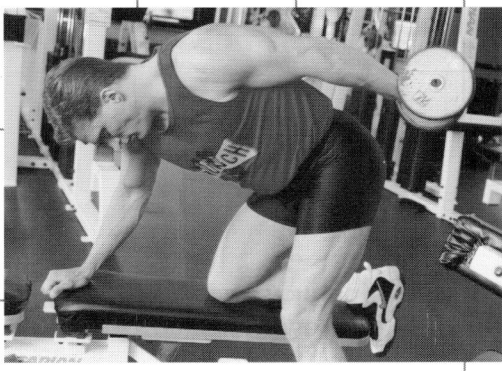

BEGINNER'S LUCK

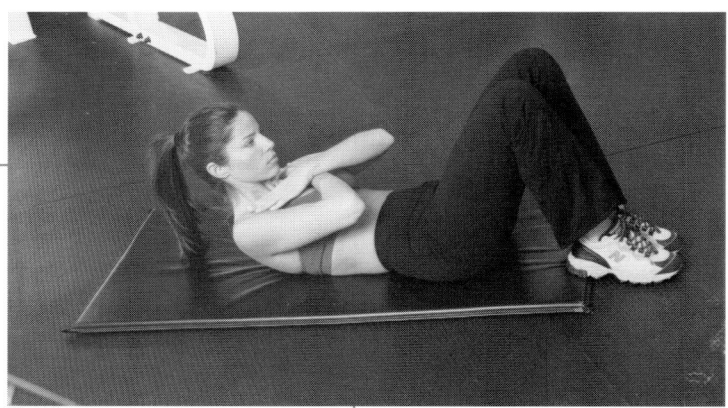

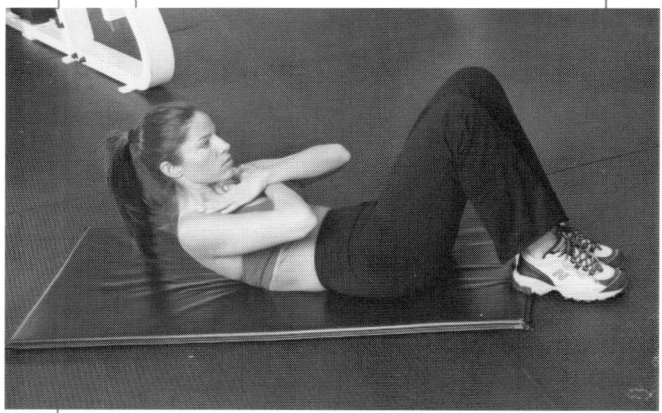

STANDARD CRUNCHES

Lie on your back on the floor with your knees bent up and your feet flat on the floor. Cross your hands over your chest. Do *not* interlock your hands behind your head-you can pull on your neck and injure yourself. Crunch up, bringing your head toward your knees and slowly lowering it again- but not all the way to the floor! Keep your shoulder blades just off the floor. Do not crane up— think of sliding toward your pelvis and shortening the distance between it and your rib cage.

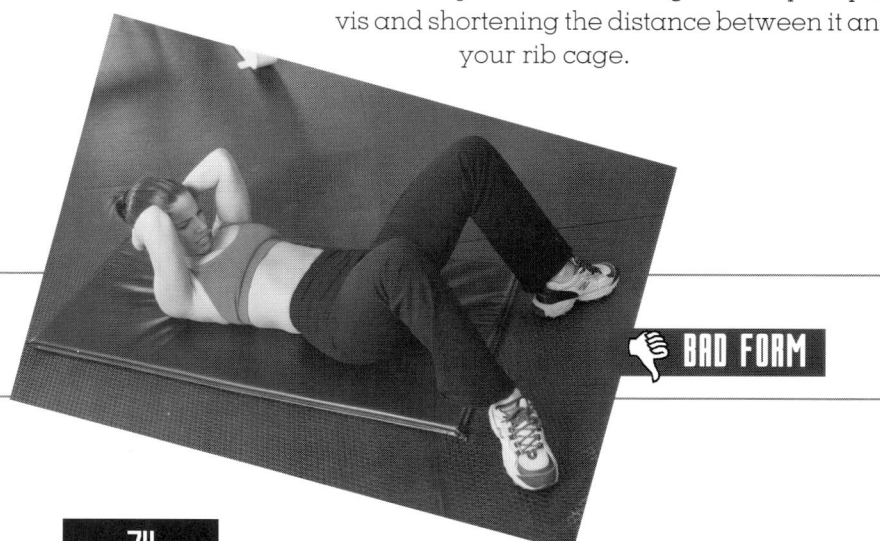

BAD FORM

CRUNCH VARIATION #1

Assume the same starting position as the first crunch, only bring your feet off the ground, so that your calves form a 90 degree angle with your thighs. Bring your head to your knees while keeping your feet off the ground and your legs level. Do *not* cross your ankles—doing so can pull your lower back.

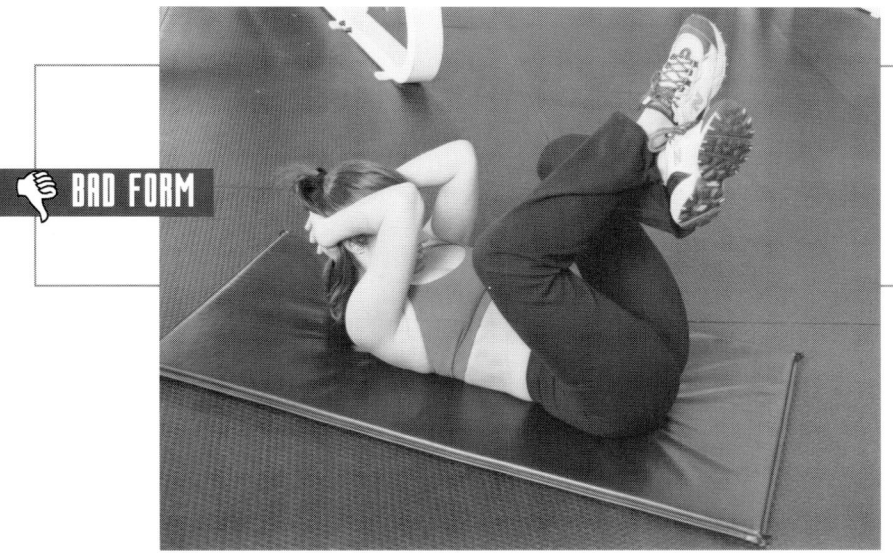

BAD FORM

CRUNCH VARIATION #2

Same as the first variation, only place your hands at your ears, with your elbows out to the side, and bring your knees in to your middle as you crunch your upper body.

BEGINNER'S LUCK

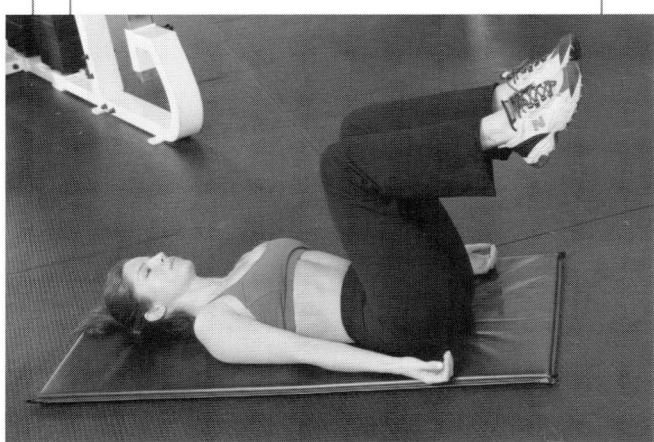

REVERSE CRUNCH

Take the same position as the standard crunch, only place your arms flat at your sides with your palms up. Raise your pelvis and lower again. This crunch works the lower portion of your abdominal muscle.

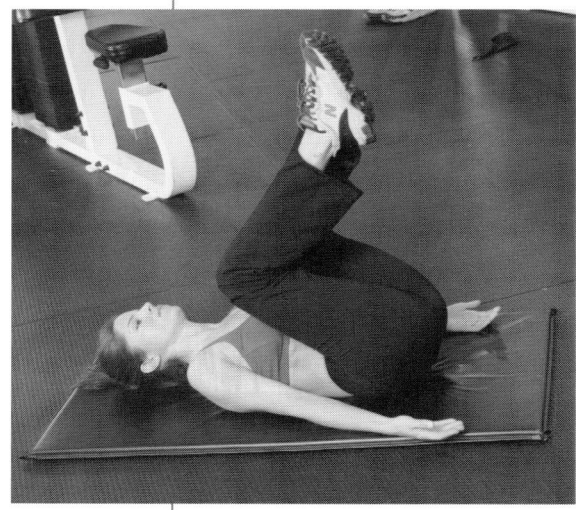

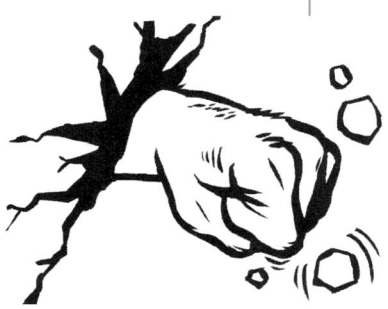

CRUNCH FITNESS

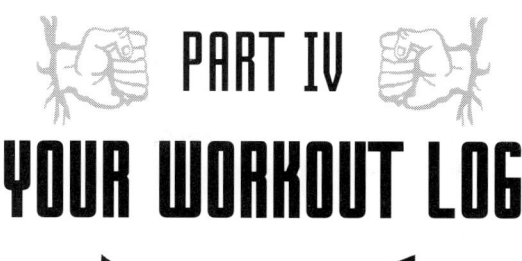

PART IV
YOUR WORKOUT LOG

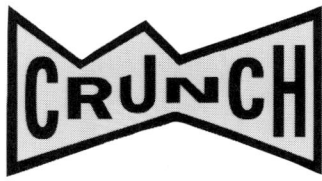

Keeping a fitness log is the best way to appreciate the changes your body is going through and how well your workout is working for you.

Here is a sample of a beginner's log sheet for one week:

WEEK # 3

Date: *1/12*
Days of the week I worked out: (M) (T) (W) (Th) F S (S)
Lifetime goal: *Achieve a consistent level of fitness and health*
Date goal is met:
Long-term goals:

Work up to two sets of each exercise on weight training days by 3/1.
Bike continuously for 40 minutes (from my house to beach and back) on cardio days.
Lose 10 pounds in five weeks (by 2/22).

Weekly goals:

Bike continuously for 25 minutes (from house to post office and back) on three cardio days. (1/18)
Complete one 15-rep set of each exercise on weight training days. (1/18)
Complete one set of each ab crunch each weight training day. (1/18)

Warm-up

Type: *jumping jacks*
Time: *5 minutes*
Stretching: *I can finally reach my toes doing the pike stretch!*

BEGINNER'S LUCK

Cardiovascular training

Type: *Biking*

Time: *20 minutes Monday, 25 minutes Wednesday and Friday*

Distance: *To Wilson's and back on Monday. To the Post Office and back on Wednesday and Friday. Couldn't face the hill before the post office.*

Target heart rate: *130 bpm*

Strength training

Exercise	Sets	Reps	Weight
Leg press	1	15	10 lbs.
Leg extensions	1	15	10 lbs.
Seated leg curls	1	15	10 lbs.
Squats	1	15	8 lbs.
Push-ups	1	10	
Machine chest press	2	15	10 lbs.
Pull-ups	1	10	40 lbs. assist.
Seated machine row	1	15	10 lbs.
Barbell curl with body bar	1	15	8 lbs.
Seated overhead tricep extension	1	15	5 lbs.
Standard crunches	1	10	
Crunch variation #1	1	10	
Crunch variation #2	1	10	
Reverse crunch	1	10	

Notes

I notice I don't get as tired climbing the steps to my fourth-floor office. I've been sleeping really well, and waking up refreshed. My jeans are starting to feel a little looser around the waist.

Use the log sheets in this section to track your progress, and photocopy pages to use when you run out. Or, make up your own fitness log. Be sure to review your past accomplishments from time to time.

YOUR WORKOUT LOG

WEEK

Date:

Days of the week I worked out:

Lifetime goal:

Date goal is met:

Long-term goals:

Weekly goals:

Warm-up

Type:

Time:

Stretching:

Cardiovascular training

Type:

Time:

Distance:

Target heart rate:

BEGINNER'S LUCK

Strength training

Exercise Sets Reps Weight

Notes

YOUR WORKOUT LOG

WEEK

Date: _____

Days of the week I worked out: _____

Lifetime goal: _____

Date goal is met: _____

Long-term goals: _____

_____
_____
_____
_____

Weekly goals: _____

_____
_____
_____

Warm-up

Type: _____

Time: _____

Stretching: _____

Cardiovascular training

Type: _____

Time: _____

Distance: _____

Target heart rate: _____

BEGINNER'S LUCK

Strength training

Exercise   Sets   Reps   Weight

Notes

YOUR WORKOUT LOG

WEEK

Date:

Days of the week I worked out:

Lifetime goal:

Date goal is met:

Long-term goals:

Weekly goals:

Warm-up

Type:

Time:

Stretching:

Cardiovascular training

Type:

Time:

Distance:

Target heart rate:

BEGINNER'S LUCK

Strength training

Exercise   Sets   Reps   Weight

Notes

YOUR WORKOUT LOG

WEEK

Date: _____

Days of the week I worked out: _____

Lifetime goal: _____

Date goal is met: _____

Long-term goals: _____

_____

_____

_____

Weekly goals: _____

_____

_____

_____

Warm-up

Type: _____

Time: _____

Stretching: _____

Cardiovascular training

Type: _____

Time: _____

Distance: _____

Target heart rate: _____

BEGINNER'S LUCK

Strength training

Exercise   Sets   Reps   Weight

Notes

YOUR WORKOUT LOG

WEEK

Date: _____

Days of the week I worked out: _____

Lifetime goal: _____

Date goal is met: _____

Long-term goals:

_____
_____
_____
_____

Weekly goals:

_____
_____
_____
_____

Warm-up

Type: _____

Time: _____

Stretching: _____

Cardiovascular training

Type: _____

Time: _____

Distance: _____

Target heart rate: _____

BEGINNER'S LUCK

Strength training

Exercise	Sets	Reps	Weight

Notes

WEEK

Date: _____

Days of the week I worked out: _____

Lifetime goal: _____

Date goal is met: _____

Long-term goals:

_____
_____
_____
_____

Weekly goals:

_____
_____
_____
_____

Warm-up

Type: _____

Time: _____

Stretching: _____

Cardiovascular training

Type: _____

Time: _____

Distance: _____

Target heart rate: _____

BEGINNER'S LUCK

Strength training

Exercise   Sets   Reps   Weight

Notes

YOUR WORKOUT LOG

WEEK

Date:

Days of the week I worked out:

Lifetime goal:

Date goal is met:

Long-term goals:

Weekly goals:

Warm-up

Type:

Time:

Stretching:

Cardiovascular training

Type:

Time:

Distance:

Target heart rate:

BEGINNER'S LUCK

Strength training

Exercise	Sets	Reps	Weight

Notes

YOUR WORKOUT LOG

WEEK

Date: _____

Days of the week I worked out: _____

Lifetime goal: _____

Date goal is met: _____

Long-term goals: _____

_____

_____

_____

_____

Weekly goals: _____

_____

_____

_____

_____

Warm-up

Type: _____

Time: _____

Stretching: _____

Cardiovascular training

Type: _____

Time: _____

Distance: _____

Target heart rate: _____

BEGINNER'S LUCK

Strength training

Exercise	Sets	Reps	Weight

Notes

YOUR WORKOUT LOG

WEEK

Date:

Days of the week I worked out:

Lifetime goal:

Date goal is met:

Long-term goals:

Weekly goals:

Warm-up

Type:

Time:

Stretching:

Cardiovascular training

Type:

Time:

Distance:

Target heart rate:

BEGINNER'S LUCK

Strength training

Exercise   Sets   Reps   Weight

Notes

YOUR WORKOUT LOG

WEEK

Date: _____

Days of the week I worked out: _____

Lifetime goal: _____

Date goal is met: _____

Long-term goals:
_____
_____
_____
_____

Weekly goals:
_____
_____
_____
_____

Warm-up

Type: _____

Time: _____

Stretching: _____

Cardiovascular training

Type: _____

Time: _____

Distance: _____

Target heart rate: _____

BEGINNER'S LUCK

Strength training

Exercise   Sets   Reps   Weight

Notes

CRUNCH FITNESS

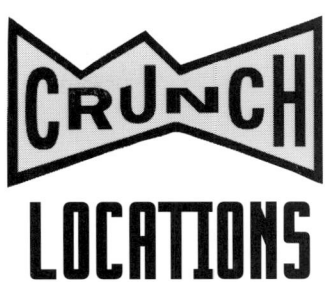

LOCATIONS

Where to work out, pretend to work out, or just stand around calling our personal trainers "Hans" and "Franz" under your breath.

NEW YORK CITY

404 Lafayette Street
(Astor Place and 4th Avenue)
212.614.0120

54 East 13th Street
(University and Broadway)
212.475.2018

162 West 83rd Street
(Columbus and Amsterdam)
212.875.1902

623 Broadway (at Houston)
212.420.0507

152 Christopher Street
(at Greenwich Street)
212.366.3725

1109 Second Avenue
(at 59th Street)
212.758.3434

144 W. 38th St.
(7th Ave. & Broadway)
212.869.7788

LOS ANGELES

8000 Sunset Blvd.
(West Hollywood)
323.654.4550

SAN FRANCISCO

1000 Van Ness Avenue
(Geary and O'Farrell)
415.931.1100

MISSION VIEJO

The Kaleidoscope Center
27741 Crown Valley Parkway
949.582.8181

MIAMI

1259 Washington Avenue
(South Beach)
305.674.8222

CRUNCH LOCATIONS

ATLANTA AREA
[ALL LOCATIONS: 800.660.5433]

Crunch Club Cobb
North by NW Office Park
1775 Water Place
Atlanta, GA 30339

Crunch Roswell
Roswell Exchange
11060 Alpharetta Highway
Roswell, GA 30076

Crunch Gwinnett
Gwinnett Prado
2300 Pleasant Hill Road
Duluth, GA 30136

Crunch Buckhead
3365 Piedmont Road, Suite 1010
Atlanta, GA

Crunch Town Center
Main Street Shopping Center
2600 Prado Lane
Marietta, GA 30066

Crunch Stone Mountain
Stone Mountain Square
5370 Highway 78 South
Stone Mountain, GA 30087

TOKYO

Crunch Omotesando
4-3-24 Jingumae Sibuya

Coming soon to Las Vegas and Chicago!

Visit us on the Web at
www.crunch.com

CRUNCH FITNESS

Have questions about this workout?

Ask the authors at:
WWW.GETFITNOW.COM
*The **hottest** fitness spot on the internet!*

FEATURING...
"Ask the Expert" Q&A Boards
Stimulating Discussion groups
Cool Links
Great Photos
Full-Motion Videos
Downloads
The Five Star Fitness Team
Hot Product Reviews
And More!

**Log on today to receive a FREE catalog
or call us at
1-800-906-1234**

Fit Test / Personal Training Session

15% OFF! 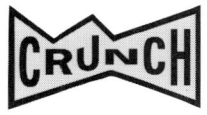 15% OFF!

IT'S EASY ... Come into any CRUNCH location and receive 15% off your first purchase of personal training. Then just sign, date, and present this coupon at the fitness desk to set up your session.

_____   _____
MEMBER NAME   SIGNATURE

_____   _____
TRAINER NAME   TRAINER SIGNATURE

_____
DATE OF SESSION

Cannot be combined with any other offer. Valid for one use only

---- CUT AT DOTTED LINE ----

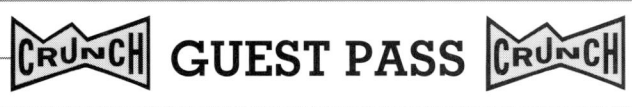

$22 value!

Must show picture ID to use facility.
The same guest may use only two guest passes per year

_____   _____
MEMBERSHIP REP   EXPIRATION DATE

OUR MISSION AND PHILOSOPHY

We at CRUNCH warmly welcome people from all walks of life,
regardless of shape, size, sex, or ability.
People don't have to be flawless to feel at home at CRUNCH. We don't care
if our members are 18 or 80, fat or thin, short or tall, muscular or mushy, blond or bald,
or anywhere in between. CRUNCH is not competitive, it is non-judgmental,
it is not elitist, it does not represent a kind of person.
CRUNCH is a gym; a movement which is growing as we continue to perfect our ability
to create an environment where our members don't feel self-conscious,
and don't worry about what others think.
At the heart of CRUNCH's core stands a tremendously experienced and energetic staff
dedicated to creating an environment where everyone feels accepted—
a truly unique place!

WWW.CRUNCH.COM

The **hottest** fitness spot on the internet!

OUR MISSION AND PHILOSOPHY

We at CRUNCH warmly welcome people from all walks of life,
regardless of shape, size, sex, or ability.
People don't have to be flawless to feel at home at CRUNCH. We don't care
if our members are 18 or 80, fat or thin, short or tall, muscular or mushy, blond or bald,
or anywhere in between. CRUNCH is not competitive, it is non-judgmental,
it is not elitist, it does not represent a kind of person.
CRUNCH is a gym; a movement which is growing as we continue to perfect our ability
to create an environment where our members don't feel self-conscious,
and don't worry about what others think.
At the heart of CRUNCH's core stands a tremendously experienced and energetic staff
dedicated to creating an environment where everyone feels accepted—
a truly unique place!

WWW.CRUNCH.COM
*The **hottest** fitness spot on the internet!*

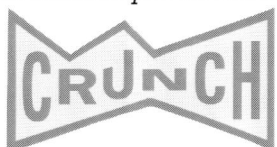

------ CUT AT DOTTED LINE ------

NEW YORK CITY

404 Lafayette Street
(Astor Place and 4th Street)
212.614.0120

54 East 13th Street
(University and Broadway)
212.475.2018

162 West 83rd Street
(Columbus and Amsterdam)
212.875.1902

623 Broadway (at Houston)
212.420.0507

152 Christopher Street
(at Greenwich Street)
212.366.3725

1109 Second Avenue
(at 59th Street)
212.758.3434

144 W. 38th St.
(7th Ave. & Broadway)
212.869.7788

LOS ANGELES

8000 Sunset Blvd.
(West Hollywood)
323.654.4550

SAN FRANCISCO

1000 Van Ness Avenue
(Geary and O'Farrell)
415.931.1100

MISSION VIEJO

The Kaleidoscope Center
27741 Crown Valley
  Parkway
949.582.8181

MIAMI

1259 Washington Avenue
(South Beach)
305.674.8222

ATLANTA AREA
(All locations: 800.660.5433)

Crunch Club Cobb
North by NW Office Park
1775 Water Place
Atlanta, GA 30339

Crunch Gwinnett
Gwinnett Prado
2300 Pleasant Hill Road
Duluth, GA 30136

Crunch Town Center
Main Street Shopping
  Center
2600 Prado Lane
Marietta, GA 30066

Crunch Roswell
Roswell Exchange
11060 Alpharetta Highway
Roswell, GA 30076

Crunch Buckhead
3365 Piedmont Road,
Suite 1010
Atlanta, GA

Crunch Stone Mountain
Stone Mountain Square
5370 Highway 78 South
Stone Mountain, GA 30087

TOKYO

Crunch Omotesando
4-3-24 Jingumae Sibuya

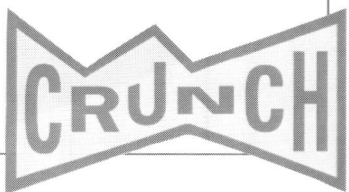

CHICAGO AND LAS VEGAS COMING SOON!